Emotional Recovery from Workplace Mobbing

A guide for targets and their supports

By Richard Schwindt M.S.W., R.S.W

To be tested is good.
The challenged life may be the best therapist.
Gail Sheehy

Table of Contents

First Aid

You may be in the midst of emotional turmoil when you read this so I am going to start with a quick set of principles for healing from workplace mobbing. There is more to this book but if you are in crisis this is a place to start. Most of this advice is helpful whether you have left work or remain exposed to workplace aggression.

Take care of your physical health.

People who are mobbed frequently suffer from sleeplessness, stomach problems, dizziness, nausea and headaches. They really are sick. Over time, they may become very sick as serious illness emerges from the chronic stress. If you are still exposed to the mob you are under siege. Your body is going to remain in "fight or flight" mode, which is characterized by a high state of emotional and physiological arousal. Good sleep, good food, lots of exercise, hydration, avoidance of drugs (including excess caffeine, alcohol, prescription drugs) are critical. Enlist your health care provider right away.

Make yourself an expert on workplace mobbing.

Mobbing is a well understood phenomenon. You need to be prepared intellectually in order to face the workplace and understand the dynamics of mobbing. From a survival point of view, the phenomenon is predictable. Reading about workplace mobbing for the first time can be overwhelming and painful. That said, you are stronger afterwards for the experience. Others may not understand what is going on but now you do. This confers many advantages. But be wary of bad advice in the anti-bullying literature. Advice to confront aggressive people, remain locked in anger and use HR processes will usually make things worse. One of the critical questions you want to ask is: should I fight back? Make an informed decision. There are excellent resources listed at the end of this book.

Gather your real supports around you.

You cannot do this alone. Part of the problem is that you are becoming isolated at work. That is part of the strategy; leaving you alone, confused and angry. Then you can be more easily discredited. You may not have supports at work. People who you think are supports may be working against your best interests. It is wise to share little, even to those you think of as friends at work. It is more important that you have supports outside of work. Depending on how far the mobbing process has gone you may have alienated friends and family. Be frank with them, take responsibility for your actions, tell them you want to get better and need their support. You may need to have friends and family on board. This isn't something you want resting on one overwhelmed partner alone. You need to understand that despite the horrific things going on at work the world is full of good people.

Respond on the High Road

You might try fighting fire with fire; using underhanded and bullying techniques. I would advise against this. For one thing it is not likely to work and for another it is antithetical to healing. Mobbing is driven by malice and fear; neither of those emotional states are going to help you. Something you will read in the literature is that there is no "winning" for the target. A healthy target will not so much "win" as move forward as a better and wiser human being. But you can lose. You may lose your job, trust, self esteem, colleagues, health and well being. Playing dirty, humiliating others is one of the ways you lose.

"Do unto others as you would have others do unto you"

Some version of the Golden Rule exists in most cultures, religions and philosophies and psychologist Martha Stout notes that it remains: "the most succinct and clearly operationalized moral philosophy ever conceived."

Understand that we are mind, body and spirit.

Under stress we become detached from ourselves. We lose our ability to be mindful. We zone out with television, food, drugs, whatever is available. Mobbing targets may lose their sense of humour and forget what it is to laugh. When they are at work, or even at home with loved ones their preoccupation with the mobbing puts them somewhere else. The world narrows until there is just that ugly fear staring them down. Part of recovery is rediscovering our richness. Whether we go for a massage, enjoy a good meal, spend intimate time with our partner, pray, look at the beauty of the day we will realize that we are much more than our work.

Position yourself spiritually for change.

Remember that this is a book about healing. All healing comes from a deeper place. A belief there is higher authority, whether God or Goddess or simply a humanistic belief in the need for human beings to act decently in a challenging world can help people to carry on when their world is falling apart. Someone who cannot find some form of truth, goodness or morality, or fails to see it, will not be able to heal.

Understand how people heal emotionally.

Much of this book is devoted to the *process* of emotional healing. It is a beautiful and innate gift that is ours to discover. And it is astonishing that there are so many ways to heal. Yes, sitting down with a therapist helps. But that is just the tip of the iceberg and every good therapist understands that. There are as many approaches to healing as you can imagine.

Preface to the 2018 paperback edition

A few years ago I was interviewed on the topic of workplace mobbing for the Kingston Whig Standard and made the cover of the Saturday edition. The following Monday one of my clients came to her session and told me she had gone into her boss's office and slapped the newspaper down on his desk.

That would be a strange thing to do with an eReader, so now you have the opportunity to slap this book down on the boss's desk, though I wouldn't recommend it. **Emotional Recovery from Workplace Mobbing** has been a success; it outsells all my other (19) books put together. It has sold well, but, more importantly, I have heard from people all over the world, and in dozens of occupations, that the book helped them survive and heal.

While originally written in 2013, it has held up well so I have left this edition more or less intact. I am sorry you have to read this. I hope it helps. And remember - I know this better than anybody - you are not alone.

Richard Schwindt, June 2018

Introduction

Emotional healing usually begins with our story; our narrative. Mine might go like this: I am a man, a husband, father, grandfather, social worker, writer, artist and psychotherapist. I try to do my best to be a good person and help others but I am imperfect. I experienced a workplace mobbing that devastated my life. I broke down. I had a stroke. I recovered physically and emotionally with the help of many others. I am grateful for all that I have received. I made a decision to use my skills as a writer and therapist to help others who had similar experiences. That decision was healing too.

The field of workplace bullying and mobbing remains problematic on many levels. Some fundamental concerns have not been addressed fully, or are difficult or awkward to address:

Most bullying is in fact mobbing, a different way of looking at workplace aggression that does not lend itself to simple solutions.

Women are abused in the workplace approximately twice as often as men. Call me simple but to me a woman being abused is an abused woman. Yet mobbing is rarely identified as a woman's issue like other forms of abuse. I believe this is to a great extent because - unlike any other form of woman abuse - at least half of the abusers are other women and at least a third of the targets are men.

We have not confronted the reasons why mobbing more often takes place in environments with job security, unions, good pay and benefits. Mobbing can happen anywhere but Universities, Schools, Social and Volunteer Agencies, Hospitals and Civil Service offices are hotbeds.

Organization policies to address "harassment" are widely recognized by targets and advocates as worse than useless. This is because they are working from a false paradigm (individualized rather than systemic). They will almost inevitably bow to power, and those participating in investigations, tribunals, etc are compromised emotionally and physically.

Psycho-clinicians who should be addressing this issue are silent. We have not identified the concerns unique to targets of mobbing, nor have we addressed the social context from which mobbing arises. In part this may be because some of us have been mobbed or participated in mobbing ourselves.

People, who participate in the discussion, write about mobbing, and research abuses in the workplace bring their own biases and experiences to the table. That is not a bad thing but at this stage in history it can be confusing to a reader and unhelpful to anyone living the nightmare that is mobbing. To this book I bring thirty years of clinical experience as a psychotherapist, the experience of a workplace mobbing, recovering from the subsequent breakdown and most importantly the experience of many women and men who have seen my videos, read my articles and shared their stories with me.

The true innovator was Dr. Heinz Leymann (1932 - 1999). He was a psychologist with an additional academic degree in psychiatry. Leymann first began to describe the phenomenon of mobbing while investigating the suicides of nurses. He went on treat more than 1300 people in outpatient and residential settings. While much of his work has been translated into English he remains relatively unknown among North American clinicians.

Most of the work on mobbing has come from academics and advocates. Their work is terrific and their influence will infuse this book. But I am neither. I am a working therapist who sits down every week with fifteen to twenty people as an Employee Assistance Counsellor for a large company, and in my private practise. While people seek me out in my private practise based on my website and word of mouth, I actually see more targets in my EAP practise. This is remarkable given that no special effort is made to stream them my way.

I am pragmatic about my work. While I am well versed in several common approaches to therapy, I am also a full member of the Canadian Association for Clinical Hypnosis (Ontario Division), and have experienced a number of alternate approaches including spiritual and energy approaches. I believe that emotional recovery can come from many places and what is offered by doctors and therapists represents the tip of the iceberg. Generally I am open to many possibilities for change and the shortest route to feeling better.

I am not going to share much about my own experience. There are several reasons for this. One, I have a gag order. Two, my experience is one among many and not unique. And finally, it is boring. This is an overlooked dynamic of mobbing; trying to relate their experiences targets can end up sounding petty, even to people who care about them. This is frustrating to people who cannot find the words for the nightmare they are living.

There are important acknowledgements at the end of this book. I did not accomplish anything alone. That said I want to acknowledge up front the influence of several people who have supported and inspired me. They include Journalist, Anton Hout; Sociologist, Dr. Kenneth Westhues and Anthropologist, Dr. Janice Harper. However, I am entirely responsible for the content herein and any misrepresentation of their ideas. In my clinical work the sources of learning and inspiration are too many to mention, including my teachers and clients. Emotional healing and psychotherapy represent a large and complex field; this represents my take on the subject. For example, I go into some detail on CBT (Cognitive Behavioral Therapy) and Hypnotherapy. This is not because these are the best approaches to therapy but simply because they are approaches I use on a regular basis. And, as you will see, there is much more to the story of healing. Finally, I do use a few case examples in the book. They are a mix of different cases and distorted beyond recognition.

What is workplace mobbing?

"Mobbing", which University of Waterloo Sociology Professor Kenneth Westhues describes as the *"stressor to beat all stressors"*, is a viral phenomenon: *"normally carried out politely, without any violence, and with ample written documentation. Yet even without the blood, the bloodlust is essentially the same: contagion and mimicking of unfriendly, hostile acts toward the target; relentless undermining of the target's self-confidence; group solidarity against one whom all agree does not belong; and the euphoria of collective attack."*

Dr. Gary Namie describes bullying as: *"repeated, malicious, health-endangering mistreatment...psychological violence, a mix of verbal and strategic assaults to prevent the target from performing work well."*

INTRODUCTION

In his WAMI (Waterloo Anti-Mobbing Index) Westhues adds:

"No two cases are alike, but mobbing typically proceeds from subtle, informal techniques of humiliation and exclusion to overt and formal measures." Five stages are commonly distinguished:

Avoidance and ostracization of the target.

Petty harassment: making the target's life difficult.

A critical incident that triggers formal sanctions: "something has to be done".

Aftermath of the incident: hearings, appeals, mediation.

Elimination: target quits, retires, is fired, becomes disabled, dies of stress related illness, or commits suicide."

Although not evident from the quote, Gary Namie and Kenneth Westhues are coming from a different place. The difference between individual and group aggression in the workplace is crucial to understanding a rift in the field. Gary Namie is likely the best known individual in the American anti-bullying movement and Kenneth Westhues is well known for his many articles, books and presentations on mobbing. Bullying and mobbing are not versions of the same phenomenon; they are different and imply different mind sets and responses. For me as a clinician the mobbing paradigm represents the accurate description of what actually happens in the workplace and is therefore more useful in subsequent healing.

As Janice Harper has pointed out "bully" has become a stigmatizing term that is used to identify someone as bad or abusive and then to justify punitive acts towards them; in other words, mobbing. I haven't entirely thrown the word out because most people, confronted by an abusive individual at work use that term. And there are people driven by malice who do reprehensible acts. The problem is that "bully" is easily enlisted to describe anyone who is disliked or targeted. It then becomes meaningless as a descriptor. Harper also points out that workplace struggles are not about issues but power and emotion. The moment someone takes someone's side a group dynamic comes into play.

This dynamic is progressive and can escalate into a form of workplace aggression directed against an individual, using all the tools of normal management practise and many creative augmentations. As a mobbing progresses logic goes out the window and is replaced by an implicit "might is right" ethos and a ramping up of emotion and fear. This is an occult process where the increasing exclusion of the target from organizational activities, gossip and rumour leaves them isolated. They will almost certainly be abandoned by their closest friends and supports. Tactics include spreading rumours, the more outrageous and implausible the better. As the pressure on the target builds there is commonly a critical incident, usually a visible error at work or emotional outburst. This serves the process of rebranding the worker as bad or mad. As unanimity builds about the worker's flaws complaints, grievances and processes may arise that embroil the organization in a formalized effort to humiliate and disgrace the target. Attempts by the worker to bring objectivity to the process or representation for themselves are met with outrage and anger. As the rhetoric becomes more inflammatory participants may begin to fear violence from the target. The target begins to fear violence from the mob. Once the target is eliminated there is significant likelihood that someone else will be targeted.

Who is mobbed?

Greg was a distinguished professor of Environmental Science with a long list of publications and a record of public service. Sarah had a mild developmental handicap and worked packing boxes in a small factory. He was being shunned by colleagues and she was being verbally abused - called "re-tard" by other workers in the factory. I saw them both in the same week. Both were unsure about how they could face the workplace again.

Anyone can be mobbed. There is no one "type" of person who is mobbed. But again, there are patterns, and we need to acknowledge that some people will be bullied or mobbed over and over again in their respective workplaces. And some people will never be mobbed. People who are identified as "bullies", including aggressive individuals, can be mobbed. There has traditionally been some virtue ascribed to targets of mobbing. And often they are virtuous people: "the nice, the vulnerable, the best and the brightest." I see all of those people; the only Christian, the only Jew, the woman who is sweet, the guy who lacks social skills, the woman who is pretty, the innovator, the woman who always looks out for her sisters, the guy who asks the wrong questions, the black person. Of course I am a therapist and always look for the best in everyone. My clients are human and I am sure many of them are not completely virtuous; perhaps even annoying or "bullies".

Carlos had taken on large property and oil interests in his home country for years. He faced down intimidation and death threats with equanimity and courage. He fell apart after his team at the office turned on him.

One clue for me is who best disappears into the crowd. Maybe that is the survivor. I also always ask myself *cui bono*? Who is doing well while this is going on? We know that friends of the target are offered privilege, comradeship and advancement. We know that a certain kind of person remains cool calm and collected while the target melts down. We know that some people are good at pulling strings. And we also know that up to 2 percent of the population are psychopathic and enjoy messing with people wherever they are. There is no perfect answer for this. What is clear is that no one deserves it; the good, bad, beautiful or ugly. And, finally, it becomes part of the workplace culture.

> *Culture eats policy for breakfast every day of the week.*
> *Peter Drucker*

In the end mobbing thrives in places where it is allowed to thrive. Certain workplace cultures permit the existence of bullies and string pullers, passive bystanders and helpless workers and identification of scapegoats.

What happens to people who are mobbed?

If you can keep your head when all about you
Are losing theirs and blaming it on you
If you can trust yourself when all men doubt you,
But make allowance for their doubting too…
Or being lied about, don't deal in lies,
Or being hated, don't give way to hating…
If you can meet with Triumph and Disaster
And treat those imposters just the same;
If you can bear to hear the truth you've spoken
Twisted by knaves to make a trap for fools,
Or watch the things you gave your life to, broken
And stoop and build 'em up again with worn out tools
If you can force your heart and nerve and sinew
To serve your turn long after they are gone,
And so hold on when there is nothing in you
Except the will which says to them, "Hold On
Excerpts from IF by Rudyard Kipling

Most of my clients eventually hear a sound file of a tiger growling and roaring in captivity. Many are rattled by the sound; it seems to speak to something deep inside us. That is the sound we have feared throughout our existence as Homo sapiens. The sound of knowing one mistake could kill us; the sound that triggered the vast array of physiological responses designed to help us run or fight. We have not changed. While we rarely run into tigers we do run into stress that triggers these responses.

The extent of damage varies. Generally it is a factor of how long the abuse lasts, the nature of the abuse and your vulnerabilities. Questions to ask yourself:

Am I sleeping?

Are loved ones noticing my deterioration?

Have I lost or gained weight?

Am I having stomach problems?

Am I preoccupied with work?

Am I anxious or scared?

Am I trying to soothe myself with food, shopping, gambling, sex, drugs or alcohol?

Is my temper frayed?

Have I lost my sense of humour?

As the abuse progresses people may feel paranoia; a loss of ability to reality check and emotions that can't be controlled, particularly intense fear, rage and suicidal ideation. People become sick; heart problems, bowel issues and muscular-skeletal issues are common. People may start to experience violent thoughts; fantasies about hurting the perceived abusers. To the extent that this happens to people who often have no previous mental health concerns it can feel dissonant and unreal. Their relationships outside of work deteriorate as they withdraw, abuse substances or continue to struggle controlling their emotions.

I counselled a woman who was under severe job stress. A manager, she seemed to always be on call; always dealing with crisis and staff problems. Fran, in her thirties, married with two small children would come home and scream at them all, then suffer terrible guilt.

She felt like she was failing everyone. And yet I could see the warm, funny and competent woman underneath. Her marriage and family life were stressed but no genuine dislike lay behind the anger. She loved her kids and described her husband as a caring man. The problem was work. Her boss was by turns harsh and undermining. Fran found that no matter how hard she worked, she achieved little except more assignments. I encouraged her to get out and find another job. With a good salary and roots at work this was difficult but the price she was paying in her wellbeing and family life had put her on the path to a complete breakdown and possibly a divorce. When she did leave her job it was a relief to everyone. Her boss was deliberately making her life difficult and ignoring the signs of impending breakdown. She had been brought in to clean house and no one looked too closely at the methods she employed.

Why do people stay in toxic workplaces?

Every stock trader knows that we put more energy into trying to recover losses than consolidating gains. Good stock traders know how to recognize losing propositions, minimize the loss - cut and run.

Why do people stay in toxic workplaces? To understand this is to address the biggest challenges of counselling targets. The most common reason is the most obvious; people need to make a living. However, there are deeper reasons that address the stubborn clinging to disaster that characterizes many targets. In simple terms they have been robbed of something and want it back. And many of them are going to try to stay until they do, no matter how quixotic the goal becomes. Sometimes they have been robbed of concrete things like raises, offices, responsibility, friends, health, mental health and privacy. Other times they have lost status, self respect, dignity and confidence. The more advanced the abuse the less likely anyone is to recover either the concrete or less concrete losses. You will likely lose more. Your biggest mistake is looking for any of these things in an abusive workplace.

It is not unusual for me to hear some version of "Why should I leave? They're the ones in violation of policy. They have no right to do this to me. I have put 10 years into this organization and I'm a good worker. I am not going down without a fight. I don't want them to win." It is impossible to argue with that. At the same time, ask yourself the cost you are willing to pay (and your loved ones) to be proven right in money, time and health. Ask your significant others. I'll bet a lot of them are saying bluntly: "get the hell out."

Good name in man and woman, my dear lord, is the
immediate jewel of their souls.
Who steals my purse steals trash; 'tis something, nothing;
'Twas mine, 'tis his, and has been slave to thousands;
But he that filches from me my good name
Robs me of that which not enriches him,
And makes me poor indeed.
Iago in Shakespeare's Othello

What kind of organizations foster mobbing?

Workplace mobbing can happen anywhere but it is no accident that the top three professions to call the now defunct National Hotline on Workplace Mobbing in Britain were nursing, teaching and social work. On the face of it this doesn't make sense. All these professionals typically work in unionized work environments with job security, pension plans, harassment policies and rules. As I mentioned earlier job security is one key; it simply isn't easy to get rid of anyone, let alone a well liked and competent employee. To evict someone from the workplace the organization has to resort to subterfuge and escalating emotional abuse. The processes, even the ones there to help, can be used to delay any real airing of thoughts and emotions, and can even be used to shift the spotlight onto the target.

> *The map is not the territory.*
> *Gregory Bateson*

These organizations neither recognize nor reward excellence. In fact, excellence in a stable environment can be viewed as a threat. The emphasis on "objective" measures, accreditation and accountability mean that liars can easily hide behind statistics and bafflegab. In a for profit organization mobbing an excellent employee happens but is more demonstrably stupid. In a public organization his eviction may be only noticed by patients or clients. The message to bystanders, attached to their job security and pensions is unmistakeable. Don't talk about it, shut down your feelings and don't stick your neck out or you are next. This is particularly cruel on bystanders who have spent their careers helping others; they may resort to denial or mental contortions to help them believe that the target somehow deserved their fate.

When the target departs there is invariably an attribution error: stress at home, a stroke or heart attack, "she walked out on us", couldn't handle the normal work stress, personality conflict or mental instability. Staff in public service organizations tend to be poorly managed by middle managers who themselves are preoccupied with placating the managers above them. Everyone is in a perpetual state of fear about unmet recording standards, impending budget cuts, "negotiations", the next accreditation and the latest reorganization.

In the end we will not remember the words of our enemies but the silence of our friends
Martin Luther King

Grieving

People who have been abused in the workplace have usually suffered multiple losses. They may have lost their confidence, well being or sense of safety. Concretely, they may have lost their livelihood, savings, home, career, friends, or health. And their process of recovery resembles grief. To lose a job is difficult; to lose it after fighting a mob is worse, leaving a gaping hole in your life. Your friends at work may have turned on you. You may have left clients, patients, or students without saying goodbye. You probably loved your job, and the people there. You hoped that your departure might be for a better job or retirement, involving hugs and warm goodbyes. And you can't get rid of those thoughts in your head, the fantasies that someone is going to hurt you, or that you will somehow get them back. You hate yourself for turning into the "mental case" the mob claimed you were. You avoid people and activities, even those that have nothing to do with your former workplace. You feel sick even when you are not sick. You may have crying spells. And who the hell are you anyway? You used to be a nurse, administrator, teacher - now what? Grieving a mobbing experience can be slowed by denial, legal or grievance processes, using mobbing behaviours yourself, entry into another mobbing situation, addiction to alcohol, drugs, gambling, sex or food. You do need to move on in your own way.

How people heal

I am going to write about some of the many tools you can bring to bear on your recovery, including some non traditional approaches, but they all begin with hope and intent. Look around your world and find someone who has recovered from some sort of serious blow. People do recover, all the time. Sure we read about being forever scarred by experience and hear about people devastated by tragedy but in simple terms we have profound gifts for healing; both innate and in the culture around us. But they can only be activated by hope and intent. People are forever changed by painful events and always remember profound losses but they can come back and move forward; living healthy and productive lives.

And so can you. Workplace mobbing does present significant challenges to healing. People I see are more like abuse victims than people who have lost a loved one to cancer or a car accident. The mobbing target has had a look into the dark side of human nature. The fact that it happened in a brightly lit office or meeting room only makes it more disturbing, compounded by the fact that people may not believe them or understand what has happened.

This book is not about advocating for yourself in the workplace or managing bullies and bystanders. This book is about managing yourself; the escalating anger, sadness, fear and de-compensation in body, mind and spirit. For self advocacy I would recommend that you have a look at **"What every Target of Workplace Mobbing Needs to Know"**, edited by Anton Hout or **Mobbed! A Survival Guide to Adult Bullying and Mobbing** by Janice Harper.

I don't want to achieve immortality through my work;
I want to achieve immortality through not dying.
Woody Allen

In most cases I think people should consider leaving their workplace. Some of my clients get lucky and something changes at work but generally it doesn't. I do not believe that people can recover emotionally while remaining exposed to abuse. For people who remain in any abusive context we are more talking about survival. As a therapist I have to take a stand for people's emotional health. I want you in a safe place where you are respected and honoured for who you are and can therefore heal. I would venture that your loved ones would agree with me. In my experience people want their family members out. Here are some reasons why people remain in abusive workplaces:

This is the only job in my field in this town.

I don't want to let down the clients/kids/patients.

This is wrong and I am going to fight back.

I don't want them to win.

I only have a year left until I get my pension.

My husband is unemployed.

The Union says they will help me.

I have friends at work who are going through the same thing.

If I keep my head down this will go away.

The company has a policy against harassment.

I've made a complaint to the Human Rights Commission.

We will lose medical and dental coverage.

I'm not the bully here.

Remember, in the end, remaining in a mobbing situation even for the best of reasons will probably lead to illness, financial loss and emotional breakdown.

For those who do stay I recommend a few things; some of which are mentioned at the beginning to the book. For example, therapist, Glynnis Sherwood in her article in **What Every Target Needs to Know** recommends that targets take a page from the repertoire for supporting abused woman and prepare a safety plan. I have made this recommendation to many of my clients for two reasons; it makes practical sense and it provides some psychological security for people who fear that remaining in the workplace will become unbearable. What is in a good safety plan?

Your most recent resume

Websites and other resources for finding jobs.

An updated financial plan, including all assets and liabilities.

A list of things that could go out the window in case of financial hardship.

If you have a pension, an update on its status.

People you could call on in an emergency.

Places you could move to if necessary.

Friends and family members with special skills that might help you.

Distinguish between poor and healthy, versus sick with a disability pension. Also distinguish between real and perceived hardship. People who have been twenty years in a secure job with a pension may be shocked to discover that people live without these things. Also, in a consumer society it is striking how much money goes out to things we really don't need (how much do you spend on cable and lattes?)

Here is a list of things that people might say if you ask them how they changed:

I went for counselling and my therapist helped me to see how the people at work preyed on my need to be liked.

I felt the Holy Spirit enter my body and began to understand that prayer and faith in God can really help.

I was introduced to a drumming group that had just started up on the Rez. When I began to understand my culture I began to understand myself.

My painting (writing, singing, dance, drumming, stand-up comedy) is what stands between me and going crazy.

The medication helped me to focus enough to find another job.

Once they began to treat the diabetes I felt strong enough to make a decision.

I got together with others who had been mobbed. We went to our MP and demanded that the government investigate the abuse of workers in our community.

At my lowest point I decided to volunteer for the Soup kitchen and you would not believe how good it was to forget the mobbing for awhile and focus on someone else.

When I finally finished night school and got a job as a teacher I was able to walk away from the abusive workplace with my head held high. It's amazing the difference having some choices makes in this world.

I decided to stop drinking. I needed to face what happened with a clear mind.

I sat down with my wife, apologized, and then we really talked. She understood far more than I realised.

Once I decided that a job wasn't worth dying for, the rest was easy.

It turns out the guy I talk to every day in the coffee shop teaches Tai Chi. I'm starting his class tomorrow.

I put it out of my mind.

The problem just went away.

There are as many possibilities out there as you can imagine. Most hurt is immoral (e.g. abusive boss) or amoral (e.g. painful illness). Moral and ethical acts on the other hand lift you in mind, body and spirit. So while the last 2 points are morally neutral, the others are ethically forward looking and involve positive intent.

The four horsemen of self care

I do yoga, I do Bikram and I run, and I eat really healthy.
Lady Gaga

A few years back I attended training with the Canadian Society for Clinical Hypnosis taught by Dr. Max Shapiro, a leading hypnotherapist and psychologist from Yale University. It was a great two days but I was struck by his insistence on asking each client four questions on their physical self care: Are you sleeping? Are you eating properly? Are you getting exercise? Are you staying hydrated? He was clear that without self care the techniques in his arsenal would be useless. The need to take care of ourselves under stress is obvious and yet, now that I have incorporated them into my practise I see how often they are neglected. They represent the low hanging fruit of healing. Targets deteriorate physically as well as mentally when they are mobbed and often let these things go. I see people in a high state of physiological arousal (stressed). Self care activities should de-stimulate as well as maintain wellness.

Of all these activities sleep is perhaps the most problematic for targets. The common scenario is some poor guy who wakes up at 5 am, looks at the clock and starts worrying about the work day. Maybe other workers are waiting with some new degradation. Maybe he is thinking about how he will handle his workload. Or maybe he is just too scared to go. Most people claim to understand the basics of sleep hygiene even if it is not practised. At the core is your need to de-stimulate in the hours before bed and use the bedroom only for sleep and sex. So no workout tapes, spicy vindaloo, espresso, Metallica tapes or Vin Diesel movies at the end of the night and especially in the bedroom. Leave your Blackberry in the den. This much so obvious. So obvious in fact that people who try all this stuff, throwing in some sleep medication, and still don't sleep get freaked out. They are convinced that they are going to turn into walking zombies. It helps to get your head to equate rest and sleep and learn to enjoy the quiet hours. You can reframe your state: why not lay there, rest and let your brain off the hook for a bit. You might try meditation, self hypnosis, or just lying there doing nothing.

Self hypnosis 101 (a simple sleep technique)

Become aware of your breathing; try counting your breaths up to ten and down again. Or reversing "breathe in, breathe out" to "breathe out, breathe in".....

Be aware of the support the bed is giving your body and the pillow your head...

Put your mind in each toe, then each foot then your ankle and work your way up....

Give yourself the explicit message that all sounds inside and outside the bedroom are helping you to rest and the only sound that matters is the sound of your inner voice....

Imagine your favourite kind of flower; in your mind's eye, look at it, smell it, touch it and imagine the sound a breeze might make as it brushes by. Now change the flower and see how it looks in another colour or with other flowers....

Introduce a mantra or phrase; it should be positive because the message will be going directly to your unconscious mind (e.g. "God's Peace" or "Quiet Rest")

If it helps, write down what you plan to worry about before you go to bed and consider the job done. Fatigue is a common outcome of mobbing and can show up for many reasons. It can be a symptom of depression or other illness, or the body's natural need to shut down after sustained stress. You should be staying tight with your medical provider through all of this so do bring it up with her. If things are unmanageable she might consider sending you to a sleep lab or providing medication. De-stimulate in any way you can and as a friend - herself a former target of workplace abuse - put it to me, enjoy the rest.

Exercise is critical. It is the easiest call in health care. Most evidence suggests that walking does the trick for most people. This is one reason I prefer my clients to own dogs. It's a riff on the old joke: If you want a friend at (name your organization) buy a dog. If it was practical I would invite your dog to the session and tell him to guilt trip you to walk. Nonetheless I am suspicious about some of the more extreme forms of exercise. The endorphin happy-chemical thing associated with extreme workouts can be quite stimulating and\or depleting. If you are considering taking up triathlons or punching sandbags have fun but it might not leave you in a calm state. On the other hand Tai Chi, Qui Gong, Yoga, or Swimming settles your body on a deeper level.

If there is ever a big meeting of targets there should be a workshop called: did you lose or gain 15 pounds? Chances are you did one or the other. We don't eat normally when we are messed up. In a state of high arousal I cannot eat and found myself over a few months in the minus 15 camp. Many of my clients confess to binging on junk food for the salty\sugary\fatty respite. When I see diabetics under stress their sugars are all over the map. Never forget that mobbing is potentially life threatening and though forests have been felled for books on good nutrition you will need to monitor your intake. The four horsemen come ahead of everything else in your response to the efforts that have been made to destroy you as a human being.

By the way, need a drink? No, not that kind, wait for the section on addictions. No, I mean water, milk, juice, electrolyte stuff, tea. People get dehydrated and don't know it. According to the Mayo Clinic website:

"Water is your body's principal chemical component and makes up about 60 percent of your body weight. Every system in your body depends on water. For example, water flushes toxins out of vital organs, carries nutrients to your cells and provides a moist environment for ear, nose and throat tissues."

It goes on to say that we can become hydrated from both liquid and food sources men need roughly 13 cups of liquid and day and women, 9. In the end it is not far from the eight 8 ounce glasses of water we have been hearing about for years.

Agency and Communion

People come to see me about things to do with work, school, family or some form of internal struggle. Generally I apply my counselling skills on their behalf and we work together towards some kind of goal. The success of this process depends on many things; most of them taking place outside my office but important among them are the ideas of agency and communion. This is an idea from health care. We need a sense of our ability to influence events around us. Without this we deteriorate. One of the keys to understanding this concept is that we never have complete control of anything in this world but we need the capacity to influence events.

This is an important distinction for targets. You will not be in control of events at work. In fact, attempts to control the work environment may make things worse. What you may be able to influence is your own response to events and how you choose to manage your life. Communion refers to your engagement in a loving and trusting way with others. By others I mean people outside of work. This is essential for emotional survival and recovery. I worry more about an isolated client than one surrounded by family and loved ones.

Factor X

Leave all the afternoon for exercise and recreation, which are as necessary as reading. I will rather say more necessary because health is worth more than learning.
Thomas Jefferson

With my clients I call this factor X for a few reasons. It sounds vaguely cool and I don't really know what else to call it. I could call this dimension hobbies or interests but it runs deeper than that. We are complex beings and there is something about the extra dimension that enriches our lives and serves as a protective factor against emotional decompensation. These are things that can fall by the wayside under the extreme stress of mobbing. _I do not consider them luxuries but essential components of healing._

I love artists. People who paint, draw, sculpt, write, dance, make music, do stand up comedy, arrange flowers or cut faces out of wood with a chainsaw have an ability to express what is inside their heart. With real artists it is also a need that moonlights as therapy. For many people emotional turmoil aids in the creative process. Their work can help heal others. If you know anything about stand up comics you know there is little chance of them being held up as models of mental health. My own personal favorite, Jeremy Hotz (the funniest human being) will be on my list of acknowledgements as the only person who could, in my worst moments, transform me from despair to convulsions of laughter.

Many of my clients love to hike in the woods or ski. There are beautiful parks nearby. I have lived for the past 25 years in areas where hunting and fishing and other outdoor activities are accessible and popular. Urban areas have parks and gardens that can fulfill the same need. Engagement with a natural setting is health promoting and takes us out of the sickness of work.

The benefits of athletic activities speak for themselves. Individual sports are great, as are workout routines. Team sports such as hockey, baseball, soccer are particularly helpful. They are generally social, take place outside of home and work, and are physically beneficial. I still hold my reservation that certain activities (e.g. external martial arts, power lifting) can be over stimulating but the woman who plays soccer with the girls (who don't work with her) on Tuesday has a leg up on the one who is home alone with a bottle of white wine and Dexter on Netflix.

For most of our human existence spirituality has been indistinguishable from healing. I include all forms of spirituality in this account, including principled humanism and ethical atheism. Spirituality takes you to a higher place; a place where you begin to understand the temporary nature and pettiness of the agony from work. Spiritual People have access to shared worship, prayer and caring communities.

Evidence based therapy

A chicken and an egg are lying in bed. The chicken is leaning against the headboard smoking a cigarette with a satisfied smile on its face. The egg, looking a bit ticked off, grabs the sheet, rolls over and says ... Well, I guess we finally answered "THAT question!"

Rigorous research has been done on the process of psychotherapy, going back decades. I have found reading evidence a valuable adjunct to my engagement with clients, reading literature and philosophy, establishing my own healthy core for practice, and exploring the natural and quantum world. The establishment of evidence in the world of psychotherapy and emotional healing is complicated and controversial. Left to many organizations, "evidence" somehow constitutes simple proof that there is only one way to proceed. The principle problem with this thinking is best put by the authors of the introduction to the widely respected Bergin and Garfield's handbook of Psychotherapy and Behavior Change:

Though many practitioners and the public may be comforted by the notion that they are offering or receiving an empirically supported psychotherapy, the fact is that the success of treatment is largely dependent on the client and the therapist, not the use of "proven" empirically based treatments. Proof of effective treatment needs to be based on measurement of treatment responses rather than provision of the "right" treatment.

This has enormous implications for emotional healing of any kind. American psychologist Scott Miller has stated:

Over a thousand studies have demonstrated that the alliance between the clinician and the client is 7 times more important than the technique of the therapist. And the largest source of change (accounting for at least 40%), virtually ignored by EBP (evidence based practise), is accounted for by what the client brings—their strengths, struggles, culture, and preferences. The approach accounts for so little of change, while the client and the practitioner—and their relationship—account for so much.

In practise this means the therapist must be able to form a positive and trusting relationship, see the client as a resourceful human being and identify those resources.

She must listen carefully to the client's evaluation of the helping experience and modify her approach accordingly; what Miller would call "Practice Based Evidence".

Moreover, this set of principles applies to any helper; not just professionals. Psychotherapy is one small piece of comprehensive healing. Healing cannot neglect the spiritual, political and cultural context of human beings. There is nothing wrong with using "evidence based" approaches. They will likely work for the same reason that any other approach works. But be wary of any approach that limits you and especially any approach that seems more about the approach than your personal issues.

Welcome to the healing bazaar

When inspiration does not come to me,
I go halfway to meet it.
Sigmund Freud

The conventional position on seeking help for mobbing is often that you engage your family doctor and perhaps a therapist. There is nothing wrong with that but why limit yourself? People don't do so in the real world. They go looking in all kinds of strange corners for assistance. Do they run into quacks? Of course. And if you want to stick to people who are accountable to professional standards do it. I'm just telling you that there is more. Here is a list of possibilities. I have divided the healers into four categories but remember that there is overlap and no rule saying that you cannot check out multiple sources of help. It is, however, courteous and smart to let the people helping you know who else is in the picture. Good helpers want to complement each other or at least not interfere with or contradict someone else's work.

The professional healers

There are many excellent therapists of all professional backgrounds who can help you but at the same time most operate under a handicap. While she will likely have sound clinical skills she will not likely have the training or even access to the training necessary to understand the organizational dynamics at play, how an otherwise strong individual has been ground down, and the realistic obstacles faced by targets. She might not challenge your decision to stay. She may urge you to use HR and Union supports without understanding the risks that accompany that path. Worse, she may urge you to confront a "bully", an approach that can easily lead to escalation of abuse.

A **Psychologist** normally has a doctorate in Psychology and registration as a Psychologist in their jurisdiction. Some specialize in Psychological testing and research but many are excellent therapists. They are on the expensive side but partially covered in most insurance plans.

Psychiatrists are what many people inexperienced with therapy think of first. As medical specialists they are responsible for medical units and psychiatric programs and many specialize in diagnosis, serious mental illness and medication. It can be quite difficult to find one without a referral, though when you do they are often covered under insurance or provincial health plans. It is more difficult to find one who specializes in psychotherapy, though when they do they are often excellent.

Many **Social Workers** have extensive training in psychotherapy and do it every day. They are cheaper than psychologists, more available, and who you are likely to run into if you are seen in a social agency or an EAP program. More and more they are covered under insurance and extended health plans. Recent changes have also classified them as "medical" for the purposes of tax deduction in Canada.

Historically the term **Psychotherapist** has had no precise meaning and could be used by anyone. In Ontario that has changed and it has a precise meaning now, given to people who belong to the new Ontario College of Psychotherapy, along with people like **Nurses**, people with **Masters level training in Psychology**, **Occupational Therapists** and **Clergy**. The three professional groups mentioned above can all call themselves psychotherapists.

While many grumble about **Family Physicians** doing psychotherapy the truth is that much of their day is occupied doing therapy on the fly. And they have the added advantage of knowing the medical issues and having prescription rights. There are some who do specialize in delivering therapy.

The physical healers

I'm thinking here of people like acupuncturists, massage therapists, chiropractors, naturopaths and others who practice forms of healing that directly involve your body. Even looking at my short list here there is considerable differences in education, outlook and the nature of their work. Any of the above for example might treat anxiety, which has many physical manifestations. Some may be special individuals who seem to have gifts of insight and touch. It is worth finding out who they are. If you have become an active agent in the healing bazaar you will investigate, ask questions and figure out what works for you.

The spiritual healers

Historically spiritual healers have done more actual healing than any other group you can name, regardless of their group, sect or denomination. While this category embraces some charlatans the spiritual dimension of healing is often ignored by professionals. There are traditions of healing in all the major religions. Christians may have prayer services, Islamic people may consult with the Koran, Wiccans may cast healing spells and indigenous people may use sweat lodges and shaking tents. Principled atheists draw on larger principles of how we coexist with our fellow human beings. That said, any principle can be distorted. In the context of an abusive workplace, lies and the need to bow to power will result in people using ethical principles to justify terrible acts. That this has happened throughout human history doesn't so much belie those principles as speak to how people acting in groups can be manipulated.

The financial healers

From the spiritual to the pragmatic, we run across the issue of money. This is the glue that holds many targets to toxic environments. As mentioned before, mobbing environments often have excellent pay, benefits and job security. People in those environments feel safe taking on mortgages and debt. They expect to stay for the long term and work towards a pension and retirement. Similarly, people in single industry towns or with few marketable skills may feel hopelessly rooted in place. Faced with the loss of income many people are inclined to panic and shut down, thinking that life as they know it will fall apart without that regular paycheck. This issue comes up over and over again in the treatment of mobbing targets. These are real concerns; most of us need to work and maintain an income but money needs to have a proper discussion, not a flat out: "I could never leave my job" reflex response. Remember, people can die of mobbing and many more are disabled physically and emotionally. If you are headed in that direction ask yourself again if that particular paycheck is worth it. It is worth noting as well that many mobbing targets are bright and versatile workers who would shine in any environment. Could your concern about money reflect a loss of confidence constructed in the workplace? What price do you put on happiness? You might want to check that one out with the people you love. They may surprise you and let you know that your health and well being means more to them material things. Finally, do you have a carefully thought out financial plan that identifies your net worth, assets and debts. No? Then you are not making an informed decision. I am always struck by bankers I know or counsel telling me that the most satisfying part of their job is helping out people who are struggling. They care about what they do. Consider making a financial advisor part of your recovery team.

Social Agencies

By social agencies I mean not-for-profit organizations funded through charitable or governmental sources. These include hospital departments, adult and children's mental health programs, women's shelters, and a wide range of organizations that address mental health, addictions, family and life issues. While social agencies all have harassment policies few have any idea of the extent to which their clients are affected by mobbing. They don't know the questions to ask or recognize mobbing when they see it. Prior to widespread understanding of spousal assault, abused women were counseled for marital problems and neurotic behavior. Unless the nature of abuse is spelled out and the dynamics widely dispersed and understood it is simply not recognized, no matter how obvious it appears in retrospect. Add to this that people are being mobbed in many social agencies. When highly placed people in an organization don't want mobbing addressed or understood it can be difficult to discuss at the client level. Twenty years of preoccupation with management process has taken much of the "human" out of the "human services" but there are still good workers doing their best to help you. It will fall on you to educate them and if you've done your homework and on your way to mobbing expertise you should be in a position to help them. If you are thinking that I have things backwards just bear in mind that much of what workers do to help clients involves recognizing and amplifying their strengths and existing resources. If you, the client, are prepared to engage in a mutual working process with your counselor the chances of moving forward are increased dramatically.

Employee Assistance Programs (EAP)

Much of the counseling done in Canada and the United States is provided by EAP providers. These are private organizations that are hired by the company you work for to provide support for various issues and counseling services. The services are generally confidential and the content and the records inaccessible to your employer. Also, the services are normally short term with a component to help with crisis. Many advocates have concerns about the allegiance of EAP organizations given that their funding comes from employers. And in most cases EAP counselors can do little to advocate for their clients. That said, I work for a large EAP organization and experience no interference in my work with targets, nor do I fear for their confidentiality.

Medication

Exercise usually scores as high in evidence of efficacy as SSRI anti-depressants (not the only class of anti-depressant but the most commonly used) in mild to moderate depressions. Most therapists note the efficacy of therapy while pointing out the absence of unpleasant side effects and the acquisition of skills that can be used over a lifetime. But sometimes taking medication is helpful. I am not a doctor and do not recommend medication to people. That said, I ask everyone I see about the meds they take and send many clients off to discuss that option with their family doctor. Their responses vary from:"Wow, there are drugs for this!" to: "I would never violate this temple with chemicals from the pharma-industrial complex." I am a pragmatist and in favor of the shortest line between the problem and the recovery. Some people in the grips of severe depression or anxiety can swallow a pill when they can't do much else.

The meds are not going to change the mob but they may help you cope. Do your homework and talk to your doctor. Anti-depressants are not addictive but they have some side effects and many have withdrawal issues. Benzodiazepines (lorazapam etc) do provide some short term relief - it may even be helpful to take one before a difficult meeting - but they are also risky for long term use, a bad combo with an alcohol habit, and can be addictive. For most people they are not the first resort but it's good to know they are there if you need them.

You're Brain and you're Mind

*Where wisdom reigns, there is no conflict between
thinking and feeling.*
Carl Jung

I have mentioned the recording of a tiger roaring in
my office that I sometimes play to clients. Some shrug it
off but many experience a shiver of fear. This is a preface
to my bit on evolutionary psychology. Homo Sapiens have
been around about 200,000 years in our present form and
in less sophisticated forms millions of years before that. Our
being anything other than hunter gatherers only goes back
roughly 12,000 years. So for most of human existence our
biggest fear was animals (sabre toothed tigers really did prey
on humans) and violent neighbors. If you made a mistake
you were killed or eaten. We still have the physiology of
the creatures that had to spend a lot of time fleeing and
killing predators.

In simple terms this evolutionary heritage is
why our adrenal system leaps into high gear when the boss
confronts and humiliates us in a meeting. Our bodies want
to jump up and either run away or attack but we have to sit
there and take it. It is unhealthy and excruciating. Similarly
our emotions exist for good reasons and these to have to
be suppressed because every target knows that showing
emotion carries risk. Women, in evolutionary terms, had to
stay calm enough to make milk to feed the next generation
but they run greater risk of illness from internalization
of projected hostility. Men and women are also going to
perceived differently when they express emotions. Angry

women may be viewed as a threat and men who show weakness or emotion become more vulnerable. They are then perceived as easy targets.

Part of our current survival is understanding how our brains and bodies work in order to manage them in the face of non violent hostility. Anything that helps us manage stress is beneficial. But at the same time flowing into and experiencing our mood is healthier than fighting and internalizing it. This is not caving into rage or rumination. Pounding walls or writing 85 pages of angry rant will only flood you. But the message that *"you are not right,"* being received from all corners of the workplace needs to be directly engaged. Writing can be valuable within a disciplined context, like the exercises used in Cognitive Behavioral Therapy, or sober recording of facts. Perhaps writing a new resume that speaks to our strengths or planning a fitness routine. Similarly, our right brain will be filled with imagery and emotion; creating an alternative reality but at the same time risk feeding our primitive terror. Healthy right brain activities include knitting, drawing and thinking happy thoughts about sex. All our thoughts go directly to our bodies (so the happy thoughts on sex may need to wait until after the staff meeting).

John was a professor of medicine on the vanguard of evidence based practice. He was a hypnotherapist and had recently brought an advanced diagnostic tool from France. Instead of respect and curiosity he experienced ridicule and harassment from his colleagues. University administration began to see him as a threat to the institution and succeeded in ousting him. Even after he fled the University he was publicly attacked in the prestigious medical journal, The Lancet. Fortunately John was able to take back his life, pursue his agenda and in time his innovations were accepted.

YOU'RE BRAIN AND YOU'RE MIND

John Elliotson (1791 - 1868) was a pioneer in the use of quinine and hypnotherapy. The diagnostic tool from France was called a stethoscope. Thanks Kenneth Westhues for retrieving this story from J. Milne Bramwell.

We have a conscious mind, an unconscious mind and to some, a higher consciousness. To be a hypnotherapist is to be doomed to a lifetime of people asking if you make people quack like a duck. Moreover, to be a hypnotherapist is to hear: "my fear of heights just disappeared this week so the hypnosis last week was a waste of time." But I shouldn't complain. Directly addressing the unconscious mind has changed my whole conception of therapy. Once you understand the role of the unconscious in our lives it explains much about our behaviors and actions. Here are some of the *Prime Directives of the Unconscious Mind*, compiled by John Tozeland:

Store and organize memories

Keep you safe

Control and maintain perceptions

Seek pleasure

Run the body

So in practise this means that you are driven more by forces within - and yet part of the real you - than you realize. Moreover, these forces lie outside your awareness. Your perceptions are taken in through your senses, organized and responded to from a place of past experience, maintaining safety and seeking pleasure. Your unconscious mind will remember when you were hurt or bullied as a child and seek to protect you from current threats. It will know and respond, ahead of you, when occult (hidden) threats are at hand. It is literal, has perfect memory and therefore may respond with the tactics of a child to threats (that time you lashed out).

The most important thing is that while your unconscious response may be wrong or maladaptive it comes forward with a genuine intent to do what is best for you. While hypnotherapy directly addresses the unconscious mind much of what happens in other forms of therapy achieve the same. Reframing, changing narratives, challenging assumptions and addressing core beliefs all will influence your unconscious mind and therefore your actions and mood.

Approaches a psychotherapist might take

While there are literally hundreds of approaches to therapy mentioned they mostly work for reasons that lie outside the actual model. When you see a therapist the process will generally follow a time tested format.

Assessment and development of rapport. When you meet a therapist they want to get an understanding of what is going on and engage you in a trusting and ethical process. Therapy can be personal and intense; you will need to know that the therapist is skilled, experienced, ethical and is open to your experiences. Poor therapists place you into a predetermined mold, and the best are fluid; moving with you and your needs. Early in the session they should ensure that you understand the boundaries of confidentiality. In most jurisdictions work is confidential provided there is no threat to safety of self or others, or risk to a child under 16. In Canada therapists and files can be subpoenaed by a court. In mobbing cases confidentiality is paramount; many targets fear that people at work will discover yet another of their vulnerabilities. In most situations I would say approach a counselor who has some understanding of the situation or concern at hand. However, since counselors with good knowledge of workplace mobbing are rare I will say find someone who is open to your help and input.

Development of intent and goal setting. As I have mentioned many counselors like specific goals and I lean more towards articulation of intent. This will help guide the process. It will be helpful for you to bring to a session. It doesn't have to be anything fancy:

I just want to tell someone objective what happened.

I just want to feel better.

I don't understand what is happening to me.

I have to figure out a way of getting back to work.

I feel scared all the time.

I don't know who to trust anymore.

My husband is still upset with me and I don't know what to do.

You can elaborate and build on any of these points. Remember that goals and circumstances change. It is common in therapy for circumstances to change from session to session; your therapist should be able to flow with the changes.

Creating and acting on strategies for Change. This is where your therapist might draw on a particular model or approach. This gives him a framework for change. Be sure to provide him feedback as to whether his particular approach is helping or not. Therapy can be uncomfortable or challenging but it is seldom creepy. It can focus on past, present or future but your therapist should be able to explain why he is pursuing any particular avenue for change. You should leave the session with much to consider, new perspectives and possibly homework. There is work involved in the process of change.

Evaluating progress as you go and deciding when to end therapy. While some therapists do long term work and EAP therapists often do very short term work, research suggests that most of what is accomplished in treatment takes place in the earlier sessions. Good therapists are always trying to determine if their input is helpful and adjusting their approach if it is not. If at all possible, termination of counseling should be a mutual decision and the door should remain open should you require further help.

Cognitive Behavioral Therapy (CBT)

> *People don't just get upset.*
> *They contribute to their upsetness.*
> *Albert Ellis*

CBT, an amalgam of Behavior Therapy and Cognitive Psychology, has been developed over the past thirty years into a well researched, commonly used and accessible form of psychotherapy. I find it helpful for targets that are looking for tools to help them manage those extreme emotions that they experience. I don't see CBT as better than any other form of therapy but its prevalence allows us to examine it as a good example of the therapeutic process.

My CBT joke...

A man is driving in a remote area at night. It is late, around 3 am. Suddenly he gets a flat tire. He stops, looks in his trunk and finds a spare tire but not a jack. Looking around him he notices a farmhouse on a hill. He thinks that the farmer might have a jack and starts up the hill intending to ask him. As he walks he is thinking: " The farmer is not going to like being woken at 3 am. It's pretty embarrassing being in this situation. The farmer will probably think I am an idiot from the city and start chirping on me. That will be humiliating. Things will get worse. The farmer will get mad; he'll be yelling and screaming, the dog will be barking, I'll be humiliated and then he probably won't give me that jack".

The man knocks on the door.

The farmer opens the door and asks: "Can I help you?"

The man says: "I don't want your goddamn jack".

Most of my clients have been forced to hear that joke at one time. I like it because it so clearly illustrates the core principle of cognitive therapy. Life throws things at us every day; good, bad or horrible, but it is not the events themselves that create the emotions but the tendency of our thoughts to escalate from straightforward and reasonable to a place of distortion. Sure the farmer might not like getting up at 3 am (mind you we don't know for sure he isn't already up) but will it really turn into a crazy conflict with a barking dog? That's *possible* but it is a distortion. Furthermore, is there some sort of rule that the driver has to feel humiliation in those circumstances? It wouldn't be a good thing if the farmer got mad but why would it follow that the driver need to experience any particular emotional response.

We have stories that define our lives. Your work story might be: "I am a good worker. I care about people and doing my job well. I believe that my boss and co-workers are good and work relationships are based on trust". This works well for you. You have friends, do good work and make a wonderful addition to your organization. Then the mob; in the complex escalating series of events that define mobbing, change your story. Suddenly you are being told that your work is bad, people don't like you, and you aren't giving enough, *what made you think you could do this work at all?* With each violation you are injured: your self esteem, your health and your relationships are damaged. Every time you are abused or someone else takes the side of the mob the wound deepens. You ruminate over everything until you become obsessive. You feel a deep need to tell your story and be believed.

Those thoughts stay with you after you leave. *What did I do to deserve this? Why did my friends abandon me? Will I ever work again?* You may even have extreme and disturbing thoughts of harming yourself or the aggressive people in the workplace. Every time these thoughts come back, whether you are aware of it or not, they affect your mood and body. Some of these thoughts are destructive but true ("I was violated by someone I trusted") and others are possible but unlikely ("what if my boss comes to my home and attacks me?"). Either way, they become increasingly distorted and consuming. And we know that participants in a mob have no compunction about using your distress (caused by them) to demonstrate that you were crazy to begin with.

So pause here for a moment. What's going through your head? How are these thoughts making you feel? If you've been mobbed I might have triggered something. You can change these thoughts and prevent the hurt and distress they cause. The mob changed your story and you can change it back. In fact you can make it better. It will require work but the process of changing your thoughts is well understood. Most approaches to therapy address negative thinking. Most workbooks on depression and anxiety will teach you skills and formats for recording, assessing and changing your thoughts. This will help you investigate cognitive distortions and change them into thoughts that affirm and support you. Let's take the two examples:

"I was violated." Yes you were but this negative thought leads to more increasingly unrealistic negative thoughts (*"my life is over"*), and you become depressed, angry or sick. But people have been violated before; in work and other places. Many of them came back to lead healthy and productive lives. What did they do? What would work for you? Try substituting: *"I am resourceful and can heal like others before me."*

Someone from work may attack me at home. At work many people get away with cruelty and abuse. But most know that their sanctuary ends at the office door. Attack someone in the real world and there are real consequences. Try substituting: *I am safe at home but I will make my home secure and in the unlikely case that someone shows up and threatens me I will call the police.*

Find someone to sit and "witness" your story from beginning the end. This could be a therapist, a partner or someone you trust outside of work. This meets a need that most targets experience. It also begins a process of self examination. The deeper your commitment to the truth about yourself, the greater the gain. You will see the direct link between your thoughts, your emotions and physical well being.

The basic principle behind Cognitive therapy is easy to understand. Intervening between the situation at hand and your emotional response is a thought or thoughts.

Situation: the boss rejects your report.

Emotional response: you feel anger, humiliation and fear.

A CBT therapist would ask you to explore the thoughts that came to mind automatically when someone acts out of malice. So the outcome might look like this:

Situation: the boss rejects your report.

Thought: I can't do anything that pleases him. I can't handle this. I'm going to lose my job. My career is over.

Emotion: you feel anger, humiliation and fear.

These thoughts are loaded emotionally. One in particular - "my career is over"- is particularly charged or the "hot" thought. This is probably what is known as a "cognitive distortion" - a thought that is distorted to accommodate a disturbed point of view. Most cognitive distortions represent *possible* scenarios but they do not represent necessary or inevitable scenarios. Your therapist may send you off to investigate the rational basis for your thoughts and evidence for and against them. In her office or upon your return you will examine the evidence together. You may have discovered that other employers know that your workplace is dysfunctional. You may discover that outside of the reality of your workplace your reputation remains intact. You may even have discovered someone who was mobbed and yet moved on to a fulfilling and rewarding career in a safe context. Now you will be challenged to come up with a more rational thought. It might look like this:

Thought: This situation is painful but there is a world outside of this workplace. I don't want to leave and there is a real risk that I won't find work but there may also be opportunities for me.

Emotion: the negative emotions don't necessarily vanish but they may be reduced and displaced by a growing sense of optimism for your possibilities.

This approach can be particularly valuable for mobbing. People who pretend to be caring are not always supportive. They may also depend on your employer for their livelihood and reputation. You are told things that are untrue about your work. Your human flaws are grossly distorted. People lie, manipulate and get away with everything. Who wouldn't wonder what's what? And worse, you begin to look askance at the caring people. If A pretends to support you and lies, what about B? B who is supportive and caring will be hurt or wounded that you suspect them of duplicity. In the end it may not be wise to trust B either. In mobbing this is seen in the workplace but more problematically outside, among family and friends there are many people who want to support you but wonder why you turn them away. Similarly, your next workplace may be healthy and your next boss a good person but hey, you've got some trust issues now. You need to know the difference. This ability to discern the difference will only emerge over time with distance, reflection and understanding of the phenomenon that took place.

Changing your thinking does change your emotions. Moreover, CBT can be applied to any situations in life where emotions get the better of you.

Ten best ridiculous Cognitive Distortions. Could these happen to you?

I am responsible for stuff I have nothing to do with. Today it's raining. It must be me!

This guy gave me a hard time is therefore a #@!& and I am therefore a saint, or is it the other way around?

I should do this and I ought to think that; I really should!

I feel wrong therefore I must *be* wrong.

I made a small mistake; I don't tolerate mistakes so I expect the world to collapse any minute

I predict this is all going to end badly because I just *know* what she is thinking in that mean little brain of hers.

I get that my wife, kids, friends, extended family and the people I have worked with before really like me but my boss doesn't so I *must* be a terrible person.

This morning my husband said he loved me and then he hugged me, and the kids gave me a hug too and wished me a great day but I forgot to pass the peanut butter when Billy asked; they really must hate me!

Twenty people gave me a warm hello today but Bill ignored me - when did the world become such a rude place?

If I leave my job before I have a full pension it is only a matter of time until I am alone and cold, a pathetic ninety year old selling pencils in the street.

Good CBT therapists are fun and tend towards a robust sense of humor. They are present focused; not particularly interested in the past. They may exploit the absurdity of your cognitive distortions and automatic thoughts in the "C" part of CBT. In the "B" part they may have even more fun if they encourage you towards and experimental or investigative mind set. They might use exposure therapy designed to help you find a way to face frightening situations or return to frightening contexts. They may also send you out to practice social skills on strangers or ask questions of distant family members. They put you out in front of the issues, treating problems as opportunities and your emotions as the subject at hand. They understand the plasticity of the brain and know that yours can be retrained. They are like physical trainers who focus on the brain. I use stories, Youtube videos and other fun things to illustrate the ideas. Here is a story I use to illustrate CBT approaches and make a little fun of myself. Humor always anchors learning so I usually try to play it for a few laughs.

Bumping into you on the street as told to my client, Jon Green

Jon Green is my client and I tell him my CBT story. "Jon, this takes place three months in the future after you and I have completed counseling. It involves you, me and my therapist. On this day I am walking down the street, coming to the office to do a session. I am thinking about my session but feel a brush on the shoulder. I turn and see you walking away in the other direction. I continue here to do my session but I don't do a good session. Afterwards I ask myself what's wrong. Why was I so distracted?

I am self aware of my thoughts and feelings

Then I remember running into you. So why does that bother me? I think about it and come up with two explanations: one, "That Jon sure is a rude guy!" and "I must be losing it as a therapist; I did such a lousy job that Jon doesn't even want to say hello on the street."

I articulate possible explanations for my thoughts and feelings.

This upsets me and I decide that I need to speak to my therapist.

I consult with someone I trust.

I go to her office and tell her that I bumped into a client on the street and he didn't say hello, and that I thought he was either a rude guy or I was a terrible therapist. So she says to me: "Richard, are there any other possible explanations?" So I say, "Well, I suppose it's possible that they didn't see me, and it is also possible that I looked busy and they didn't want to interrupt me."

We expand the possible explanations.

"Excellent Richard; now you have four possible explanations including two that are pretty innocent. So what is the evidence for each explanation?

We examine the evidence for each explanation.

"Evidence, okay, Jon is a rude person; well he was never rude when I saw him as a client so I have no evidence. I am a terrible therapist; no therapist is perfect but over the years the feedback has been good so there's not much evidence for that. He didn't see me; well if I hadn't turned when I did I wouldn't have seen him - so there is some evidence for that. And as for not interrupting; I know I did look preoccupied so yes there is evidence for that too."

"So the evidence tends to support the more innocent explanation."

We move our support towards the explanation with the best evidence.

"Yes, but it is still bothering me."

We adopt an investigative mind set.

"Do you ever do follow up phone calls?"

"Yes."

"Why don't you phone him up and investigate what really happened today."

So I go to the phone and call you up and likely discover that you either didn't see me or that you didn't want to interrupt me..."

We have now addressed my worries effectively and decisively.

...but there is another possibility...

I pick up the phone, call you and you say: "Yes, I did see you Richard but you were a lousy therapist, didn't help me at all and I don't want to waste another minute on you. (*sound of phone hanging up*)"

Now I am devastated. I rush back to my therapist and say: "The worst was true! He was rude on the phone and I am a lousy therapist!"

Sometimes the most feared explanation is true. We can still use the process to address the new information.

"Richard, how many follow ups did you do this week?"

"Maybe ten."

"And they all told you that you did a bad job?"

"No, just this guy."

"How many have you done over the years?"

"Hundreds, thousands."

"And every week someone tells you that you are a bad therapist?"

"No."

"So why then are you elevating this guy to a point where you label yourself a lousy therapist, other than the fact that it happened today? Maybe he had a bad day or maybe you didn't do a good job. If you have the stones you could always call him back and find out but it is a cognitive distortion to give this individual the responsibility for your esteem as a therapist."

I am only scratching the surface of CBT. There are some excellent books listed in my resources list at the end of the book.

Hypnotherapy and NLP (Neuro-linguistic Programming)

> *There are more things in heaven and earth that are dreamt of in your philosophy, Horatio...*
> *Hamlet in William Shakespeare's, Hamlet*

I think of hypnosis as a powerful tool with many uses when utilized ethically by a skilled therapist. It is a natural state of mind combining both deep relaxation and focus. In that state you are more suggestible and have easier access to your unconscious mind. Most hypnotherapists will tell you that clients hypnotize themselves and that the therapist supports the process. Many therapists teach self hypnosis. Techniques can range from simple relaxation to deep regression therapy. Good therapists will answer your questions, explain the ethical restraints, address the myths (quack, quack) and make you a partner in the process. It is then used to meet the goals or intent that you have brought to the therapy process. There are few risks in hypnotherapy and they are unlikely to arise if the therapist has been properly and ethically trained.

Unlike most approaches to therapy, hypnosis has been in common usage for going on 200 years, both for physical and psychological healing. I occasionally consult a book on hypnosis that was published in 1903. Shamans understood the use of hypnosis in various forms for thousands of years before that.

I prefer hypnosis because it can do many things faster than conventional therapies and also go right to the source of unconscious struggle. When you are mobbed there is a collective effort to harm and undermine you at work and your unconscious is going to do whatever it takes to protect you; including numbing pain through alcohol, withdrawing, stimulating the fight or flight mechanism and using rage to set boundaries. The key understanding - and it is reassuring when you think of it - is that honouring the intent of maladaptive actions is a starting point to creating new behaviors more fitting to the situation. Consider checking out the Canadian Society for Clinical Hypnosis (CSCH) or the American Society for Clinical Hypnosis (ASCH) for qualified Hypnotherapists in your area.

Neuro-linguistic Programming (NLP) is also a powerful entry to the unconscious mind, without the trance state. It was developed in the 1970s by Richard Bandler and John Grinder, based on language patterning (Grinder is a linguist) and observation of some the great therapists of the time. In practical terms NLP involves visualization exercises, exploration of language use, dominant senses and associations (negative and positive anchors). Some of these exercises can be helpful in addressing the fears and anxiety that follow a mobbing. I have seen phobias become worse while someone was recovering from a mobbing and I always go to NLP first when I treat a phobia of any kind

Your workspace

I'm not talking about your *workplace*; I'm talking about your *workspace*. It is literally your space and possibly the most important space that is yours alone. You may share your home with your family but your space at work is both yours and the organizations. In NLP (Neuro-lingustic Programming) we talk about "anchors" - whether positive or negative, that associate us to places, people, concepts and things. An obvious positive anchor might be a picture of your kids. If you display it in your office it's a statement that you want the office to reflect who you are and an acknowledgement that their picture makes you feel good.

Similarly, bringing a work report into your bedroom at home is bringing a work association where it does not belong. Aggressive people will invade your workspace and violate your boundaries and this is especially true during a mobbing. If you are working on leaving an environment where you are mobbed consider moving some of your positive anchors out.

If you intend to stay and fight the mob bring in a few things that mean something to you; perhaps that somehow represent courage. During your healing process, after you have left your workplace, it will be important to know when to get rid of reminders of work. You may have documentation lying around from grievances or legal battles. Know where to keep it and when to get rid of it. I had a briefcase that a boss who made my life miserable had given me when she had (with some relief) seen me out the door. I kept it too long until one day my wife and I emptied the contents and threw it in the garage until garbage day.

If you have a new office in a new workplace, consider the process of making it your own. There may be all kinds of conscious or unconscious triggers. When I went back to work at a completely new workplace all kinds of little things set me off. I worked hard to become aware of them and identify their effect on me. One day I found myself reacting emotionally in the parking lot. I asked myself what was going on. I then realized that my new boss had backed his car into his spot; a habit shared with my old boss. It was an innocuous act but it triggered my anxiety.

By identifying unconscious triggers I was able identify the automatic thought (a la CBT) and recognize the cognitive distortions (he must therefore be like my previous boss). In my new office I moved a few things in as positive anchors. I also established some new anchors. I have always liked mint tea so I started putting a hot cup beside me when I began my first session of the day. Doing so comforted me and reminded me that I was in a place where I belonged.

Re-establishing a healthy work environment is a slow process. You will never go into a new job from a job where you were a target and feel safe right away. Wear your cross; hide a picture of the bravest woman you know in your purse. Whenever you drive by your old office yell "I'm moving on" out the car window. Have some fun; read a book on Feng Shui and remember that we are not that differentiated from our physical environment.

Eight Common Issues:

Anxiety and Depression, Addictions, Rage, Suicidal thoughts, Past Troubles, Marital and Family Problems, Paranoia

Please remember that these issues are experienced differently by different people, often overlap with other things and may pre-exist and be worsened by workplace aggression. Most emotional problems can be successfully treated and people can find growth and relief. Remember that while you may have had a pre-existing mental or physical illness, what you received is a psychological injury.

Anxiety and Depression

A cat once bitten by a snake fears the rope
Sufi proverb

Targets of mobbing go through long periods of time where they feel endangered. People at work are devoting time and energy to destroying their spirit and their lives. The primitive mechanisms of our sympathetic nervous system try desperately to protect us. The result is catastrophic thinking, severe stress, chronic physical arousal, anxiety and panic. No one who hasn't experienced true anxiety or panic can imagine the hellish fear that pushes you further and further away from your family, friends, work and life.

Driving by your old office, running into a workmate or even something irrelevant to all of it may send you into a panic, complete with thoughts of death and despair.

Addressing anxiety is counter-intuitive in many ways. The more fun you have fighting your anxiety; the more irreverent you become, the better the outcome. I know what you're thinking: anxiety is destroying my life; it certainly is not fun. But to succeed Mr. Anxiety counts on you taking him seriously. He cannot bear being laughed at. You say to yourself: "So I'm anxious, it's not going to kill me today, I've got stuff to do" and Mr Anxiety recedes. You say to yourself: "I got screwed around at work, woo woo, guess what - I lived to tell the tale" and Mr. Anxiety has a pout. Better still - and this is cool - Mr Anxiety cannot bear laughter and sexual arousal. You watch your favourite comedy on TV, or sneak off to bed early with your partner and Mr. Anxiety has to put a damp cloth on his head. Negative thoughts and ruminations lead directly to anxiety. Sometimes addressing anxiety can be as simple as keeping an elastic band around your wrist and thwacking yourself every time your mind wanders into negative space.

> *A dirty mind is a perpetual feast*
> *John Mortimer*

Throw the kitchen sink at it. There are some excellent workbooks in your local bookstore on managing anxiety and panic. For forty bucks you will have dozens of practical and helpful ideas. It will be ongoing work but you will get results. There are some easy to use assessments on the net (e.g. The Beck Anxiety Inventory) that will measure your anxiety and demonstrate the positive changes that come when you throw your heart into change. Here are some effective approaches. Again, this is the short list.

Threatened people never relax. So achieving deep relaxation is healing. Investigate Mindfulness, Bodytalk, Reiki, Massage, Qui Gong, or Tai Chi. All these approaches link mind and body while delivering relaxation and healing.

Also in the Eastern tradition, acupuncture can help heal and quiet your body, enabling you to relax.

Workbooks on depression and anxiety with a Cognitive Behavioural bias (most of them) will teach you how to record, organize and evaluate your thoughts to understand and modify your negative thinking.

Hypnotherapy is a powerful and natural tool for restoration of composure and calm. Any good hypnotherapist will be able to teach you self-hypnosis so you can achieve deep relaxation at home.

Exposure therapy is a time tested approach to addressing your fears and re-engaging the world. It is part of the "B" tradition of Cognitive Behavioral Therapy. Exposure is the opposite of withdrawal. It involves gradual or sudden (called flooding) exposure to things that we fear the most. There is also an approach called imaginal exposure that allows us to face down something in our minds when it is impossible to do so in reality.

A pervasive sense of fear that can take many forms. There is a book called the DSM or the *Diagnostic and Statistical Manual of Mental Disorders*, now called, DSM 5. As daunting as the title sounds it is actually quite readable and user friendly. There are challenges to the conclusions of the DSM. But if you want to know what is really meant by terms like anxiety and depression this is the place to look. If you do you will find that things like generalized anxiety, panic, Post Traumatic Stress Disorder (PTSD), and phobias fall under the larger category of anxiety. Only physicians and some psychologists can diagnose but it is good to be informed. A target of mobbing has been undermined, overtly or covertly attacked by people including those whose job was to support and protect her. She may have been lied to or her vulnerabilities exploited. This may have gone on for years and led to a constant state of worry and expectation. She would have gradually lost her ability to relax and let things go and thus remained in a state of physiological arousal. She is frightened and does have reason to be frightened. The body is constantly releasing chemicals and hormones originally designed to fight or flee from predation and attack. The mind is trying to figure out the limits of what is happening and almost inevitably overshoots.

When anxious, these thoughts and resulting feelings, whether they are acute and overwhelming like a panic attack or ongoing and pervasive like generalized anxiety, are exaggerated and unreal. Why has this happened? First, some people are more prone than others. This may be due to a family predisposition, a past trauma or perhaps a medical condition like congenital heart disease. More importantly, in one area of your life -work- you are under covert and overt attack. You are not safe emotionally and perhaps not physically. Your body and mind are not wired to clearly distinguish where you are or are not safe. They hear the growling tiger from our human past, react, and in time it becomes difficult to stop that reaction, no matter where you are.

There are things you can do to address anxiety but serious emotional problems can be stubborn and entrenched. Think of a story you have heard of an athlete or soldier, seriously injured. This person may also have adopted a stubborn "can do" approach to their physical rehabilitation and surpassed all expectations. You will read about how they have often anchored themselves to a specific goal ("I'm going to walk my daughter up the isle on her wedding day"). By the time you are feeling able to function or free of activity you will probably have gone through a process of goal setting, hard work and study. You will have an awareness of how you are going about change. In my years as a therapist and clinical supervisor that was always one of the surest signs that therapy would succeed.

Therapist: *What is it about therapy that is making a difference?*

Client: *We started using CBT but for some reason that just wasn't working. But when you taught me how to use self hypnosis techniques to relax and I was just allowed to talk that helped a lot.*

Therapist: *CBT really works well for most people but your feedback made the difference. It is important that we use an approach that fits your needs.*

In the 1980's when Heinz Leymann was doing his original work on workplace mobbing in Sweden he diagnosed hundreds of cases of Post Traumatic Stress Disorder (PTSD) - an anxiety disorder - among targets. PTSD is distinguished from milder forms of stress reaction by its severity and length of duration. In other words, while treatable, it isn't temporary. In fact, untreated people can suffer from PTSD for decades. The main symptoms are social withdrawal, hyper-vigilance and intrusive thoughts/ images/dreams. While we tend to associate PTSD with horrific experiences like combat, assault or accidents, there is more to it.

For one thing, recent evidence suggests that prolonged exposure to traumatic events can be more harmful than single events. Also, it is difficult to predict who will get

PTSD, though it is starting to appear that people with elevated sensitivity and imagination exposed to prolonged duress face greater risk. And it's important to note that trauma is to a great extent based on perception. Outsiders may look at targets of mobbing and see that they are stressed, dealing with some frustrations, maybe hassled a little. This is the tip of the iceberg and what they don't understand is that many targets are suicidal or think they are going to die or a heart attack or stroke. And I am convinced that on the day they release the results of a large multi-year study on the effects of mobbing (assuming someone does this someday) they will discover than many targets do die at the end of a chain of events that began with mobbing. So, if we have targets who are subject to abuse day after day, think they are going to die, suffer from the physical and emotional effects of stress is it any wonder that many end up with PTSD?

A panic attack is a truly terrifying experience. And many people who experience one end up in hospital emergency wards, convinced they are having a heart attack. A social worker describing what they observed in this situation might say: "*Allison drove by her former workplace and became short of breath, frightened, agitated and sweaty. She thought she was going to have a heart attack and drive off the road.*" Allison thinks she is going to die. She starts taking routes that avoid her workplace or if the panic increases she starts to avoid going out at all. It takes less and less to bring one on and next thing you know Allison can't work or function at all.

The options before Allison include seeing a physician, receiving a diagnosis and being directed to psychotherapy or prescribed medication. A physician would also be best positioned to rule out a genuine heart problem or perhaps some other physiological issue. And let's not forget that we are not necessarily talking about an either/or situation. There can be mental and physical sources for any emotional problem.

These are mood disorders and that includes depression. When I thought back I was surprised at how few actual depressed people I had seen in the classic sense. Typically clients I see them are anxious and highly aroused. And yet if I dig deep enough into the history of clients I treat for depression I often find childhood bullying or workplace mobbing, along with traditional progenitors like loss and trauma. There are all kinds of good resources out there on depression (see my resources section).

Here are some common indicators:

Feelings of sadness.

Feeling of hopelessness.

Loss of self-confidence.

Feeling that life isn't worth living.

Lack of energy.

Loss of interest in daily activities.

Inability to experience pleasure

Restlessness or agitation.

Feelings of shame or guilt.

Poor concentration or memory.

Change in libido.

Change in appetite.

Change in Sleep Pattern.

Most doctors and other clinicians see a lot of depression and have good skills at depression management but I want to add these considerations:

Depression can be insidious. People can slide into depression without really understanding what is happening to them. Are you aware that something is wrong? Any clinician knows the basic symptoms of depression. There is also good information available on the net. There are also good self-assessments available on the net like the Beck Depression Inventory (BDI) but they should not be used for self-diagnosis. Also they tend to score high when someone is experiencing situational stress (such as mobbing) as opposed to a true depression. What they might do for you is provide an objective indication that something is wrong.

Depression can be disguised by maladaptive behavior; forms of "self medicating", including substance abuse and high risk or high risk sexual behaviors.

Depression is as physical as it is mental; many experience predominantly physical symptoms. These can feel like flu symptoms with temperature fluxes, aches and sweats. This is one more reason why having a medical provider on the support team is important.

Depression is often experienced differently by men and women and among generations.

Like all mood disorders depression can show up when you least expect it; in other words, when "everything is going good". For the mobbing target this might months later when they are back at work or things seem to have been resolved.

Depression is correlated with suicide, cardiovascular illness and other forms of malaise. Like any other illness it can make you sick or kill you.

Depression is treatable. Yes, it can take some work but we have the technology. There are many approaches involving medication, exercise and therapy that have been proven effective.

Addictions

There is a classic joke about the habitual drunkard before the Judge in Northern England asked about why he drank as much as he did. "Your Honour" he said, "it's the quickest way out of Manchester".

There is a pattern I often see when I screen my mobbed clients for substance abuse. Every night, after work they have between 3 and 6 drinks. Call it what you like; a little too much, problem drinking, but for them it's the quickest way out of.... (Name your organization). Our brains are wired for pleasure and so is our unconscious mind. We like to feel good, which is why substance abuse is so sticky. The problem is that this is often an escalating pattern of substance use that takes away from the clarity and energy people need to survive their ordeal. Alcohol disrupts much needed sleep, subtly and relentlessly depresses mood and enhances anxiety. It also contributes to the varied physical risks you run under extreme duress. I am talking about alcohol but I could be talking about any addictive activity, including drugs, gambling, pornography, compulsive shopping, over eating, etc. People under duress may struggle with their addictive activities, and they may hear from their loved ones that they have a problem but they are inclined to say "screw it" every night and go to work taking the edge off. Once the edge is off they are likely in front of the TV aimlessly switching channels or staring into space. In other words, they have detached from the life outside of work that they need to re-engage.

People really don't want to give up their addictions until they reach an advanced stage. So what do you do? After 30 years as a therapist including seven running an addictions agency my answer is "whatever works". In the world of addictions that might mean taking either an abstinence or harm reduction approach. Both are exactly what they imply. Most people when they think about addictions treatment think about detoxification and treatment centers, intensive and perhaps confrontational modalities and twelve step programs like Alcoholics Anonymous. For many people they provide a construct that works (the disease model) as well as sober supports. And for some people abstinence is the only way they can get past the intense compulsion of their behaviors.

Abstinence doesn't work for everybody. Some people will have nothing to do with "meetings" and others can't stick with it, are phobic of social gatherings or think the paradigm is hooey.

Likewise, harm reduction isn't for everyone either. However, there are solution focused, motivational approaches that have been proven effective, and many small techniques that involve reorganizing your life, measuring and counting drinks, avoiding high risk situations etc. that will reduce the harm to your health and life.

And some people just stop. That makes clinicians look like monkeys but it is true. You do general counseling long enough and you will encounter people who just said "I'm done" and stopped.

Rage

The truth will set you free, but first it will piss you off.
Gloria Steinem

It means something more than anger. It is an intense emotion that feels overwhelming and out of control. It is difficult if not impossible to hide. It is fed by thoughts of hurt, betrayal and injustice. In mobbing situations it can torment people for years. Chinese medicine sees rage burning you up from the inside. Turned inward it can cause sickness, even death. Outwards, it can be turned against loved ones or people unlucky enough to cross your path at the wrong moment. Workplace abusers love rage and use it as proof that their underhanded actions were justified in the first place. Rage provides workplace aggressors with an opportunity to use zero tolerance or anti-bullying policies to label the target a "bully". It is exceedingly rare for targets to become violent, though in those cases the outcome is always portrayed as the mysterious act of an isolated individual who "just snapped". What's common is for targets to fantasize about violent acts; thoughts that are often disturbing in individuals who are normally peaceful and loving. I have some suggestions for addressing rage.

Acknowledge your rage honestly in a safe place (not at work!). It is common for targets to justify or rationalize the actions of the mob. Damn it, *they are working to destroy you emotionally while you are trying to make an honest living and support yourself and your loved ones.* You have good reason to be angry. You may be getting the message everywhere that something is wrong with your emotions but anger - an emotion meant to address violated boundaries - is congruent and appropriate.

Recognize that fantasy is just that - fantasy. Having a fantasy does not mean you will act on it. It is rare for someone who has not previously been violent to become violent. If you do have thoughts of acting on your anger get help.

Sit down and acknowledge to yourself that acts of rage feed into the mob's agenda and injure you further. This is part of being self aware of your thoughts and emotions.

Find a trusted person outside of the workplace that you can use as a reality check. In other words keep a source of perspective close by. Let them tell you when your rage is out of line.

Suicidal Thoughts

The idea of taking your own life is about as extreme as it gets. These feelings exist because people in the workplace have constructed a reality that claims you are the problem and you don't belong. With the force of the mob behind them this reality can be difficult to ignore. I am going to give you a counter message to consider if you ever have these thoughts and some practical suggestions for staying safe while you move forward.

You were selected by frightened and malicious people because you were somehow different. Outside of this toxic context - pay attention - you are a unique and loved individual. You have options and this feeling is temporary. You can and will heal. I'm not saying that it's easy; I'm just saying that you can do it.

Swedish psychologist Heinz Leymann postulated that 17% of suicides in Sweden were the outcome of workplace mobbing. This is an astonishing number and I have little doubt that many of them were attributed to other things (how many distressed targets have been labeled with "mental health problems"?). Some mobbed people may be vulnerable to depression but either way the emotional terrorism endemic in hostile workplaces can undermine the strongest individual.

Jill was a nurse, led bible study in her congregation, and was loved by her husband, four children and five grandchildren. One evening, after a day where no one on the ward would talk to her, she went directly down to the emergency ward and handed the triage nurse a note that said: "I am going to kill myself."

If you are feeling suicidal here are some practical measures you can take:

First, if these are just passing thoughts remember that many people have them for all kinds of reasons. Having thoughts is not the same as acting on them. They are disturbing but don't make you strange, they are a sign that it's time to make some changes.

Find someone trustworthy outside of work such as a spouse, friend, spiritual advisor or therapist. Tell them about these feelings and come up with a plan should they get out of hand (meaning that you are seriously considering acting on them). Do not swear them to secrecy; instead tell them that if should they ever believe you are going to act on these thoughts to do everything in their power to stop you.

Make a list of people or places you can call at any time. Include a local crisis number and the location of the nearest emergency ward.

Seek professional help. I don't think all our problems need professional helpers but I do for this. Doctors, social workers, and psychologists should neither be shocked nor deterred by someone's suicidal feelings. Their job is to get you to help or come up with a plan. If you feel ignored after you have expressed your concerns move on to someone else.

You have options. You always have options. Anything can be recreated, except your life.

Do I ever use guilt in these situations? You betcha. You think people would be better off without you? Think again - those who care about you would be devastated and terribly injured by your loss.

Look in the mirror and ask yourself why you are taking these cruel and insensitive people so seriously. The world is full of wonders, good and loving people. Let them control the agenda for a change. It's not time to take a life; it's time to build a new one.

Past Troubles

Children struggle with many issues, including illness, bullying, abuse and of course everything their parents struggle with, whether their parents understand that or not. As adults we are products of our past experiences. It is not unusual for example for stressed children to dissociate under severe stress; a response that can return as a stressed adult. Some people are prone to depression, anxiety and addictive behaviors. People grow up in alcoholic homes where they may learn maladaptive approaches to loyalty, perfectionism and control of their environment. Then they are mobbed. When I lived in the far north there were minus 45 degree mornings where something would break on the car. Not because I had bad cars but because the car was under stress and always had a weak link. Just like you and me. The people who mob you might figure this out and exploit it before you do. It is important that rigorous self analysis is part of your healing program.

Marital and Family Problems

Sick people and people under emotional duress often display a version of tunnel vision and can seem narcissistic in their efforts to survive the stress. In mobbing situations once you add addictive behaviors, anxiety, preoccupation with the job, and withdrawal you are no longer dealing with an ideal partner or parent. In their preoccupied state the target may be prepared to fight to the last breath. I am never above using guilt and one of my favorite questions to target intent, on staying in the fight or seeking justice is: "What does your family want you to do?" In most cases the family don't want to watch their loved one slowly going insane. If all else fails my next statement to a person intent on "winning" might be: "I know you are prepared to pay a stiff price to fight this but what price are you prepared to make your family pay?"

After four years of counseling mobbing targets I still hate telling people to consider leaving their jobs. Though occasionally something changes to make work tolerable, more often I see people wiggling on the noose only to have it tighten on them. I observe this for a one hour session but family members see it every day. Remember, mobbing targets are heir to the ills of other humans. Frequently targets end up on sick leave and family members then have them around 24/7. Family members also have to listen to long disjointed stories of the sins committed against the target at work. The fact that they are true doesn't make them less repetitive and overwhelming.

In his wonderful book, **Emotional Survival in Law Enforcement**, Dr. Kevin Gilmartin tells Law Enforcement Officers that they have to leave work and the mind set of work *at* work. In fact, they have to fully engage in family life, non-work social activities and recreation. He could have been talking to mobbing targets.

In the end your family is more important than your job and the decision about which one to sacrifice is simple. Turn the tables and nurture your spouse for a bit. Let your family know about workplace mobbing, it's place in the larger family dynamic and have the conversation you need with your partner and kids. Let them know that you don't get an exemption from being a spouse or a parent because you are being mobbed. With your kids be honest. Tell them what is going on to the extent their developmental state allows and assure them that you are addressing your stress. Kids feel their parent's stress and it effects their emotions and lives. They may be missing you, tiptoeing around you and dealing with their tribulations alone. Getting re-engaged in your family life may be the best thing you do in your journey back to health.

Paranoid

> *Just because you are paranoid doesn't mean that people aren't out to get you.*
> *Joseph Heller*

If you have been mobbed you have every reason to feel paranoid about the workplace. People *are* out to get you and feigned innocence to the contrary, most of it has happened in secret. What you don't know *can* hurt you. In my hypnosis work I have several times participated in exercises where people's muscle strength and physical abilities could be affected for better or worse by large groups sending positive or negative energy. It is mind over matter. That hostility directed your way is going to drag you down. So be as paranoid as you like. This will become a problem though once you enter the rest of your world where the ratio of the trustworthy and untrustworthy more normalized. All healthy relationships are based on trust so if you are untrusting of those who care about you paranoia will be a problem. Don't beat yourself up for it; you got that way for a reason. Just think it through, use CBT exercises and learn how to do a healthy reality check on yourself.

Jennifer's Recovery

This story, an amalgam of stories I have heard from clients, starts on Friday morning when Jennifer, once a popular manager, is met by a HR officer as she comes into the office. She is allowed thirty minutes to clear out her belongings and then she is escorted past her team into the parking lot. She has been fired. As she walks past them she can barely raise her eyes; she knows that most of them are wearing black armbands to protest her continuing employment. This is their triumphant moment.

Now Jennifer is going to recover.

Day One

What kind of shape is Jennifer in as she walks out the door? Jennifer has worked for her organization for three years and for two of those has been subject to mobbing. The aggression had escalated in the past month. Her firing is ostensibly because of her refusal to participate in a tribunal to explain her alleged "bullying" behavior; an action that was taken by management when a rumour was spread that Jennifer was demanding sexual favours from a woman colleague. That woman was never identified but she supposedly told a number of other workers that Jennifer had demanded that she meet her in a washroom for sex.

Jennifer is sick; mentally, physically and spiritually. She has lost twenty pounds and suffers from daily uncontrolled diarrhea. She has heart palpitations and her doctor wants her in for a colonoscopy right away. She would have had it earlier but her manager had loaded her with two new projects in the last month; each with imminent deadlines. Alan, her husband, is beside himself. He feels like he has lost her. All she can think about is work and all she can talk about are the various slights she endures every day. He watches her polish off a bottle of wine after work every night and go to bed. He has begged her to quit and begged her to get the medical testing. For his pains he gets screamed at and told that he isn't supporting her. She seems beyond reason. Friday night Alan calls Jeff, Jennifer's work partner. Jeff and his wife Liz have been good friends and they all went to Mexico together last year. A confused Liz reports that Jeff won't come to the phone. Alan hears Jeff yell in the background: "She brought this on herself!" Alan can barely believe his ears; Jeff and Jennifer had been best of buddies at work. Alana, Jennifer's fifteen year old daughter cowers in her room much of the time. She has stopped going out and needs persuasion from her dad every morning to go to school. She is normally smart and outgoing; her dad is terrified that she will fail her courses this year. But Jennifer doesn't seem to care. No one except Jennifer knows about the pills she has hoarded. She has a plan, if things get worse, to take them with vodka and end her family's misery. Her guilt is overwhelming.

Week one

Jennifer is like a wild animal under threat; she lies awake at night staring at the ceiling. She paces around the house; she keeps thinking about work. What are they doing? What's happening to her projects? Why doesn't Jeff call? She was there for three years; does no one care that she was fired?

She knows they didn't all feel that way. But she does get one call; from the secretary Marissa. Marissa tells her that she was a wonderful boss and that this is wrong and thanks for being good to her. After she hangs up Jennifer sobs for an hour. The next day she agrees to see her doctor.

Dr Khan insists on scheduling the colonoscopy. He also suggests that Jennifer consider an anti-depressant (which she refuses) and strongly suggests she get counseling. He recommends a social worker, Ms. Phillips. Jennifer can't do much that week. Her company has offered a settlement so Alan speaks to a lawyer. He tells them that given the settlement any action they take might involve a lot of time and work without much gain. Alan speaks to Jennifer and they agree to walk away with the money that has been offered. This feels wrong to Jennifer but she knows that she is at the end of her rope.

Month One:

Jennifer still isn't doing much. She is having nightmares every night. She knows that she should be looking for a job but she doesn't seem to have the initiative. Instead, she wanders around the mall all afternoon; just looking aimlessly in shops. She feels lost and still thinks every spare moment about work. She is scared of running into people from work and several times has ducked into a shop to avoid someone she knows.

No one has called from work but two of her old girlfriends have called and ordered her out for drinks. They weren't taking no for an answer. When she asked them, pathetically, if they still liked her they told her in no uncertain terms that they could care less about her stupid workplace; she was well out of there and they would always love her. She cried again, giggling into her Margarita.

She goes to see Ms Phillips but doesn't particularly like her; all she can talk about is her setting goals to control her drinking. She doesn't get that she really needs to drink now. Alan drags her to the bank and they meet with their personal banker who sets out a plan for them to follow. They have to skip Mexico this year but they will get by if they are careful. That said, Jennifer's parents are worried and they call to tell her that they will cover any expenses for therapy or medication. One Friday night while Alana is out at a friend's house, Jennifer and Alan make love for the first time in months. Later they take a long walk holding hands. Jennifer, a week later, goes in for tests. Shortly after, Dr. Khan calls and tells her the tests were negative and that he believes that the symptoms can be controlled through diet and stress management.

Three months

Jennifer still feels pretty messed up. She wore a holter monitor recording her heart activity for twenty four hours then met with a cardiologist who told her that she had developed atrial arrhythmia. It was mild and treatable but she would have to start on some medication and later on they might consider a surgical procedure called an ablation that is usually effective.

She never went back to Ms Phillips but she had her first panic attack in the mall; it was terrifying and threatened to keep her indoors. She called one of her girlfriends who recommended Anne; a social worker who had an office downtown. Anne was different than the other therapist. She seemed to listen and was honest; she didn't know much about mobbing but they would work together to address some of these issues and make Jennifer's priority - ending the panic - the goal.

Jennifer was greatly relieved. She began to feel like as bad as things were she might survive this. On a whim, for the first time in ten years, she went to confession. She told the priest about her guilt towards her family and shared that she had hoarded pills. When he gave her absolution he told her it was contingent on letting go of any intention of taking the life God gave her and robbing her family of a mother and wife. That made her feel really guilty. She went home and got rid of the pills. That night Alan poured a glass of her wine down the sink and blasted her; telling her what she had put her family through. The next morning she texted Alana and invited her for lunch. Shortly after a flyer came around, saying that a woman down the street was teaching yoga in her home. She went and discovered that she felt better than she had for months. The instructor knew all about "healing" and was a wealth of information. Jennifer wondered where all these good people were coming from.

Six months

Yoga is great and Jennifer doesn't think that she could get through the week without it. She doesn't feel as good about the heart meds but they seem to help. She regained the lost weight but now feels fat. One good thing; her friend who works with a volunteer group for palliative seniors wanted to develop a website for their families. Jennifer, grateful for a chance to use her brain again, took on the task. She was moved by the seniors and their families and felt like she was doing something useful.

One Sunday she received a call from someone from her old work. At first she was wary but the person on the end of the line was crying. Within weeks of Jennifer's departure the team had turned on her; the harassment had started small but now things were getting weird; she was being shunned. Jennifer feels all kinds of strong emotions welling up inside of her but she took a breath and reminded herself that was her not so long ago. She wished the woman well and gave her Anne's name. She heard herself telling the woman that there is a life outside of work. After this woman hung up Jennifer says to herself: *"it wasn't just about me..."*

Two weeks later she had a job interview but before the interview she had a panic attack and canceled on a pretense. The HR person was kind and offered to reschedule the interview. Jennifer was baffled that they would still want her but agreed. She went to Anne and Dr Khan that week. She learned some techniques to prepare for the interview and agreed to go on an SSRI antidepressant for six months. After the interview, for the first time since she left, she drove by her old office. Life with Alan and Alana was back to normal; in fact much better. They were treated pretty well while mom was unemployed; clean house, great dinners, and laundry on time. Jennifer started to think to herself; they had better not get too used to mom doing everything. Still, Alana was clearly relieved to have her mother back. They were even arguing again. God, being nice to mom all the time; *that sucked.*

One year

Jennifer still thinks of the old workplace and still has nightmares. They finally did a cardio ablation - that sure wasn't fun - then announced they had to do one more. Dr Khan agreed that she could start tapering off the anti-depressant medication now. When that was done she swallowed her pride and asked her mom for money for her and Alan to go to Mexico. Alana is slowly morphing into someone less annoying and more interested in academic success. One of Jennifer's girlfriends died suddenly this year; it was tragic and painful but she made it through with her families help. She still goes for drinks every month with her profane and irreverent girlfriends. She never went back to church but prays every night.

She has a new job, web design out of her home. She couldn't face going back into a workplace, probably ever. This means she isn't seeing Anne often but she still goes when she needs to. She heard the other day that the woman who had called her was off on sick leave; she was seriously ill. Jennifer cries sometimes. At Christmas dinner she cried when she was supposed to say Grace. But she is also laughing again, making love to Alan, being a mom and being...herself. That woman was lost and now somehow she is found

Forgiveness

You are in the midst of a mob of people acting from fear and malice. What follows for the target include sleepless nights, panic attacks, searing emotional pain, obsession, cognitive distortions, and in the worst cases, suicide or physical illness. Those who remain after the target departs are traumatized by what they've witnessed or tainted by their participation, and probably don't understand why. Forgiveness is the gold standard of healing but how do you forgive the people who create this desolation?

I plan to forgive those who mobbed me; not soon, and for some of them perhaps never, but I will strive towards that goal. Someday I may try and understand why they did what they did. But Hannah Arendt spoke of the "banality of evil" I have no desire to immerse myself in what would likely be a miserable tangle of jealousy, past wounds and fear.

I have witnessed rape victims pressured to forgive unrepentant rapists and move on. I have talked to men who beat their wives for the affirmation that eventual forgiveness provided them. I have seen people wield forgiveness like personal power to provide absolution. And expressions like, "forgive and forget" seem more applicable to neglecting a birthday than the terrible things people do to each other.

It will never be easy or quick. The dark side of targets is our shattered naiveté and deep resentment that people chose to abuse us.

But what is the alternative to forgiveness? Holding on to hate, anger, thoughts of vengeance? While anger can serve a temporary purpose, inspiring you to protect yourself and others, hate and vengeance are the antithesis of healing. They will only continue the destructive process the mob began.

Forgiveness is not reconciliation, though it would be part of a reconciliation process. Nor does it require remorse by aggressive individuals; that would simply provide them more influence over your thoughts and emotions. *In the end it is a process of letting go and moving on. Releasing you from them and them from you.*

And what of those in the workplace who resist the mob, supporting the target instead? We need to hold our gratitude for their inner compass, and honour their efforts to remain above the fray.

Gandhi said that forgiving enemies was a sign of strength and Oscar Wilde, in a different vein, noted that it was the best way to piss them off. Do your healing, and some day, when you are ready, close that door and come back fully to the world where you are loved and cherished for the special person you were meant to be.

Observations of a Therapist

Any good therapist learns from and is deeply influence by his or her clients. No matter what is written or taught we fall back on our own experiences with real people. Here are some of my thoughts:

You meet a lot of good people. Targets are not always easy to counsel but they are usually resourceful likeable people. Characteristics that made them targets often help them heal and move forward.

Counselling is usually short term. I'm not quite sure why but I usually see targets for a shorter period of time than my other clients. One theory: as people who function well in general, many targets use me more as a consultant than psychotherapist. I am fine with that. How long people come also depends on how deep they are into the experience. More exposure, more damage to fix.

Targets are usually caught up in the pain of the moment. They are preoccupied with what is happening to them. Or if they have left the abusive workplace, what has been done. Part of the clinical challenge is to remove them from that nightmare and put them back in the world where they belong.

Targets are reluctant to stop fighting and move on. This is the single greatest clinical challenge; comparable to the abused woman who won't leave her spouse.

In a society where abused women are seen as a critical concern, women abused in the workplace are ignored. Of course men are abused too but women often take the lead in labelling abuse for what it is (e.g. many abused boys receive help only when their abused sisters blow the whistle). And whoever is responsible, an abused woman is an abused woman. Workplace abuse identified as a "woman's issue" would change both the priority and sophistication of the response.

Most workplace measures to address "mobbing" are worse than useless. Some (not all) are well intended but all ignore the two reasons why tribunals, hearings and reconciliation meetings do so much harm. One, the target is usually tired and broken - in no shape to participate. Second - let's face it - in these situations might is right. And power will almost inevitably line up against the victim.

Most clinicians do not understand the dynamics of mobbing. They treat it symptomatically which is helpful up to a point but neglects the dynamics of the mob, the inner psychological experience of the client and the knowledge base on mobbing. I attribute this to a lack of training, or training that is psychologically unsophisticated or straight from the HR/policy playbook. Truth is, clinicians are mobbed too, often those who think for themselves. My field and especially my profession are doing a great impression of the "see no evil" monkeys.

In mobbing cases you can't separate the psychological from the social from the political. You need to assess and understand all of it.

Most of the situations that I see are mobbing, not bullying. The mob almost always has support from colleagues, subordinates and especially organizational leadership. Current "anti-bullying" measures have been learned, integrated and turned against the targets.

My clients have reported help from supportive spouses, organizational mentors, renegade bystanders and sometimes Unions. Rarely, I meet someone who is remorseful for participation in a mob.

Organizational leaders that truly set out to change an abusive culture would lose some superficial control but sow gains in productivity and creativity. The system is losing many of its best people. As a manager I would be thrilled to hire the quality workers who come to me for counselling as targets.

I continue to see my healers from time to time, but turning my energy towards counseling others was a healthy move for me. I have seen distressed people and some who have been made permanently ill by the abuse. That said, most of my cases have ended well. Targets are resourceful people and I have witnessed the human spirit at its best. It is, in the end, inspiring work.

Final Thought

We never wish painful experiences on people, loss, abuse or other forms of harm. And yet human beings are capable of recreating themselves better than they were before. I have seen people embittered by experiences that would seem trivial to others. I have also seen people weather grievous blows to emerge stronger and wiser. In the end there is an element of choice to whether you choose anger, vengeance and victimhood, or wisdom, empowerment and love.

Many Thanks

This may be the most important part of the book; not just because of the amazing help I have received but also the message that *we thrive on the basis of our supports.* All the people on this list helped me in small ways and large. Some of you I have known all my life; some of you showed up when I needed you.

Above all, Nina; my wife. My wonderful children, Elisa and Paul, my son in law, David and those adorable grandkids, Anna and Griffin; some for their support and some for just being themselves. Also my late father and sister, and my mother for always. Also add my remarkable sister in law, Caterina Gucciardi who was there for me at the worst moment. And to everyone else in my extended family for just being themselves.

I am blessed with wonderful friends; many of these people are professionals who brought their professional knowledge to help me but they are first and foremost friends: Christos Aslanidis, David Tate Stewart, Ellen Stewart, Janice Harper, Josh Levine, Errol Ingram, Robin Westphal, Siobhan Sexton, Kate Kroeker, Lorraine Miles, Eva Kakepetum, Brian Thomson, Julie Woit, Vince Caccamo, Susan Emery, JoAnn Ransberry, Ambrose Cheng, Christina Spencer, Gerri Trimble, Sandra Buck, Sarah Earl, Cindy Mitchell, Tricia Keen and Ron Smith.

Professionals who did their jobs with skill and compassion: Julia Laidlaw, Susan Liu, Chris Whynot, David Marcassa, Jeff Sloan, John Tozeland, and the Stroke team at Kingston General Hospital.

Millie, you are the only animal on this list but you were always there for me.

Rob Graff, you hired me when I had nowhere else to go.

Jeremy Hotz; you don't know me but you made me laugh when I didn't think I would every laugh again.

Heroes and gentlemen: Ken Westhues and Anton Hout.

People who just appeared and helped, Eric Tuttle and Rob Smith.

My clients who cannot be named but belong on this list.

Resources

This list is eccentric and incomplete but these are great resources.

Bourne, Edmund J: **The Anxiety and Phobia Workbook**, newharbinger publications inc, 2005

Burns, Dr. David D. **Feeling Good: The New Mood Therapy**, HarperCollins Publishers, 1980

Burns, Dr. David D. **When Panic Attacks: The New, Drug Free Anxiety Therapy That Can Change Your Life**, Random House, 2007

The three books listed above are terrific for understanding and addressing mood issues.

Bramwell, J. Milne, **Hypnotism, Its History, Practice and Theory**, 2nd ed., London, Alexander Moring, xvi+478 pp., 1906

Chilton, David; **The Wealthy Barber Returns**, Financial Awareness Corporation, 2012

There are many excellent books on financial planning but you can't do much better than this sequel to the classic, "The Wealthy Barber".

Duncan, Barry L., Miller, Scott D., Wampold, Bruce E., Hubble, Mark A., **The Heart and Soul of Change: Delivery of What Works in Therapy**, The American Psychological Association, 2010

To truly understand what works in therapy these guys are the best.

Gilmartin, Kevin M. **Emotional Survival for Law Enforcement: a Guide for Law Enforcement Officers and their Families**, E-S Press, 2002

I can't say enough good things about this book. Critical for police but there is much here to learn for anyone who works for a living.

Gottman, John; **Seven principles for making marriage work: A Practical Guide from the Country's Foremost Relationship Expert**, Random House/Three Rivers, 2000

Best guide I have read; very helpful. Even better, Gottman has YouTube videos where he reveals himself to be a funny and engaging speaker. I often ask couples to go home and check them out.

Greenberger, Dr. Dennis, Padesky, Dr. Christine, **Mind over Mood: Change How You Feel by Changing the Way You Think**, the Guilford Press, 1995.

This is a time tested classic for dealing with mood.

Hout, Anton (editor) **What Every Target of Workplace Bullying Needs to Know** www.overcomebullying.org

Hout, Anton (web host) www.overcomebullying.org

Anton is a great guy who makes resources people need available. Check out his site and book.

Harper, Dr. Janice, **Mobbed! A Survival Guide to Adult Bullying and Mobbing**, Amazon Kindle, 2013

Harper, Dr. Janice *"Just us Justice: The Gentle Genocide of Workplace Mobbing"* www.janice-harper.com

"Just Us Justice" is the single best article on mobbing I have read. Anything by Janice is engaging, accessible and feels true.

Lambert, Michael J (editor). **Bergin and Garfield's Handbook of Psychotherapy and Behavior Change** (fifth edition), John Wiley & Sons, 2004

Not for a day at the beach but if you want to find out what evidence based practice really means this is your book.

Leymann, Heinz *"Mobbing and Psychological terror at Workplaces,"* Violence and Victims 5 (1990)

Classic and groundbreaking article.

Namie, Dr. Gary, Namie, Dr. Ruth, **The Bully at Work**, Sourcebooks Inc., 2000, 2003

Well known book with an anti-bullying focus

Ruiz, Don Miguel; **The Four Agreements, A Practical Guide to Personal Freedom**, Amber-Allen Publishing, 2008

Ruiz loses a few people in the first chapter when he talks about Toltec wisdom but hang in, this is one book I would want every target to read.

Westhues, Kenneth; Wa*mi (Waterloo Anti-mobbing Index)* Summary for the Workplace Mobbing Conference, Brisbane 2004

Westhues, Kenneth; Preface to Heinz Leymann, *Workplace Mobbing as Psychological Terrorism: How Groups Eliminate Unwanted Members* (translated from the Swedish by Sue Baxter; Lewiston, NY: Edwin Mellen Press, 2011), pp. v-xii.

Westhues, Kenneth, *The Ouster of John Elliotson from University College London in 1838*, Commentary by Kenneth Westhues, University of Waterloo, 2009

Ken is prolific as a writer and advocate, particularly for academics. Anything by him is well written and will help you understand the phenomenon of mobbing. WAMI is a terrific and concise schema for understanding mobbing.

Wheatley, Margaret; **Leadership and the New Science: Discovering Order in a Chaotic World**, Berrett-Koehler Publishers Inc. 2006

You will not likely have read another management book like this. It is unique, wonderful and should be read by every manager anywhere.

Zanolli Davenport, Dr. Noa, Ruth Distler Schwartz, Gail Pursell Elliot **Mobbing: Emotional Abuse in the American Workplace**, Civil Society Publishing, 2005

This is an excellent book for understanding the phenomenon of mobbing.

The Author

Richard Schwindt is a social worker in Kingston, Ontario. He is author of *The Death in Sioux Lookout Trilogy*, *Dreams and Sioux Nights*, *The Love Duology*, *Social Work for Fun and Profit*, *Scarborough: Confidential*, *Sioux Lookout: Confidential*, *Kingston: Confidential*, *Emotional Recovery from Workplace Mobbing (and Workbook)*, *and six other books in the Emotional Recovery from… series*. Richard has twice been shortlisted for the International Three Day Novel Contest and won the Outstanding Book Award (self-help) for 2016 from the Independent Author Network for *Emotional Recovery from Congenital Heart Disease*. He served ten years with OAPSW Newsmagazine, two years on the Community Editorial Board of the Kingston Whig-Standard and in 2007 was second runner up in Comedian Idol of Kingston. He has been married thirty-seven years, has two adult children and two grandchildren.

www.ingramcontent.com/pod-product-compliance
Lightning Source LLC
Chambersburg PA
CBHW032115280326
41933CB00009B/857